NURSING APPROACHES TO HIV/AIDS CARE

Third Edition

By

Celia Lamke, RN, MSN, ANP-C

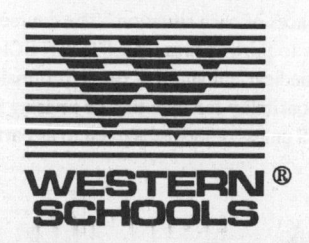

WESTERN SCHOOLS®

International Providers of Continuing Professional Education

WESTERN SCHOOLS®
7840 El Cajon Blvd. Ste 500
La Mesa, CA 91941-3617
1-619-469-2121

About the Author:

Celia Lamke, RN, MSN, ANP-C, has worked as a Primary Care Nurse Practitioner for 16 years at the Veterans Administration Medical Center in San Diego, California, where she established the medical center's HIV program. She has been a provider of health care for HIV infected and AIDS patients for 8 years and volunteers at the Owen Clinic at the USCD Medical Center. She is a member of the California Nurses' Association HIV commmittee and the San Diego County Regional Task Force on AIDS. She is certified as an HIV educator and HIV Testing Counselor by the State Department of Public Health. Celia lectures to professional and cummunity groups and has published articles dealing with HIV infection and AIDS.

About the Subject Matter Experts:

Mary A. Allen, RN, MSN, CCRN, is currently Clinical Nurse Specialist in Immunology at the Warren Grant Magnusson Clinical Center, National Institutes of Health, in Bethesda, MD. She is responsible for supporting the clinical practice of nursing staff on two inpatient units, patients of which are admitted by the National Institute of Allergy and Infectious Disease for participation in research protocols investigating a variety of immunological disorders and unusual infections, including AIDS. She is Staff Educator for the Department of Nursing. She recently completed a 2-year term as a member of NIAID Institute Clinical Research Subpanel.

Lori DeLorenzo, MSN, RN is Coordinator for the Northern Virginia HIV Resource and Consultation Center. In addition to overseeing all activities conducted in the Resource Center, Ms. DeLorenzo designed and implemented a clinical training program for health care professionals and coordinates the Resource Center's telephone consultation service. Ms. DeLorenzo has also designed, presented and evaluated numerous didactic courses related to HIV infection. Ms. DeLorenzo has a background in medical/surgical nursing and cardiovascular intensive care. She received her MSN from Johns Hopkins University and is currently enrolled in the PhD Program in Health Education at the University of Maryland.

Copy Editor: Barbara L. Halliburton, PhD
Proofreader: John Wolf, MA
Typesetter: Gwen Nichols
Graphic Artist: Kathy Johnson

WESTERN SCHOOLS' courses are designed to provide nursing professionals with general information to assist in their practices and professional development. The information provided in these courses and course books is based on reasearch and consultation with medical and nursing authoritites, and is, to the best of WESTERN SCHOOLS' knowledge, current and accurate. However, the courses and course books are offered with the understanding that WESTERN SCHOOLS is not engaged in rendering legal, nursing, or other professional advice. WESTERN SCHOOLS' courses and course books are not a substitute for seeking professional advice or conducting individual research. In applying the information provided in the courses and course books to individual circumstances, all recommendations must be considered in light of the unique circumstances of each situation. The course books are intended solely for your use, and not for the benefit of providing advice or recommendations to third parties. WESTERN SCHOOLS disclaims any responsibility for any adverse consequences resulting from the failure to seek medical, nursing, or other professional advice, or to conduct independent research. WESTERN SCHOOLS further disclaims any responsibility for updating or revising any programs or publications presented, published, distributed, or sponsored by WESTERN SCHOOLS unless otherwise agreed to as part of an individual purchase contract.

ISBN 1-878025-48-1

This book was printed using Soy-based Ink.

COPYRIGHT© 1993 WESTERN SCHOOLS, INC. — ALL RIGHTS RESERVED. No part of this material may be reprinted, reproduced, transmitted, stored in a retrieval system, or otherwise utilized, in any form or by any means electronic or mechanical including photocopying or recording, now existing or hereinafter invented, nor may any part of this course be used for teaching without written permission from the author and the publisher.

IMPORTANT - READ BEFORE PROCEEDING

Thank you for your enrollment in our continuing education course. Your WESTERN SCHOOLS Student I. D. Number and your order number can be found on the Enrollment Confirmation form which was packed with your course.

IF YOU CHOSE A MULTIPLE-CHOICE EXAM. Please read the textbook and answer the final examination questions and the course evaluation questions. The final examination questions for each chapter can be found either at the end of the chapter that they cover or in this test booklet.

IF YOU CHOSE A COURSE EXTRACTED FROM ONE OF OUR LONGER COURSES. **Do not complete the final examination questions in the coursebook.** There is an instruction sheet and a final examination in a separate test booklet enclosed with your course.

IF YOU CHOSE A TRUE-FALSE FINAL EXAMINATION. **Do not complete the final examination questions in the coursebook.** There is an instruction sheet and a true-false final examination in a separate test booklet enclosed with your course. Mark the Scantron® sheet as follows: use Choice A for True answers, and Choice B for False answers.

IF YOU CHOSE A PATIENT TEACHING PLAN ASSESSMENT. **Do not complete the final examination questions in the coursebook.** There is a separate instruction sheet for completing the Patient Teaching Plan enclosed with your course. Return the completed Teaching Plan in the envelope provided. Due to extra grading time, it will take up to one week to issue your certificate.

MARKING AND RETURNING YOUR SCANTRON® ANSWER SHEET. Each question has only one correct answer. Use the Scantron® answer sheet provided. Please mark your answers completely with a #2 pencil. Fold your answer sheet on the fold lines and mail it to WESTERN SCHOOLS in the envelope provided. **(You must mail your answer sheet to WESTERN SCHOOLS in an envelope; the form is not designed to be a self-mailer).** Your certificate will be sent to you within three working days after your answer sheet has been received by WESTERN SCHOOLS. Please include your professional license number(s) and state(s) of licensure on the answer sheet. Certificates cannot be issued without license numbers. Your certificate will include an answer key. We suggest you make a copy of your Scantron® answer sheet so you can compare your answers to the key. The key will allow you to determine your correct and incorrect answers.

PASSING SCORE. You must score 70% or higher in order to pass this course and receive your certificate of completion. Should you fail to achieve the required score, we will send you an additional answer sheet so that you may make a second attempt to pass the course.

LOGGING YOUR HOURS. Please monitor the time it takes you to complete this course and include that figure on side two of your answer sheet. A log is provided in the book to help you keep track of the hours you spend on this course. You have 2 years from the date of enrollment to complete this course. After that your file will be closed, but you may be eligible to extend your enrollment. For information please call our Student Services Department at 619/469-2121.

If for any reason you are not satisfied with the quality of our course materials, you may return the **unmarked** course within 30 days of receipt and receive a full refund (less shipping/handling).

WESTERN SCHOOLS
P. O. Box 15907
San Diego, CA 92175-5907
(619) 469-2121

NURSING APPROACHES TO HIV/AIDS CARE

COURSE LOG

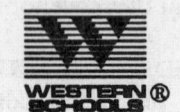

WESTERN SCHOOLS®

P. O. Box 15907
San Diego, CA 92175-5907

Please use this log to total the number of hours you spend reading the text, completing any exercises, and taking the final examination (use 50 minute hours).

Date	Hours Spent
_____	_____
_____	_____
_____	_____
_____	_____
_____	_____
_____	_____
_____	_____
_____	_____
_____	_____
_____	_____
_____	_____
_____	_____

TOTAL: ☐

Please write this number on side two of the Scantron® answer sheet.

CONTENTS

Pre-Test
Introduction i
Chapter 1 Epidemiology and Pathophysiology 1
   Introduction 2
   Beginnings and Endings 2
   HIV and The Immune System 5
   A Progression of Disease 8
   A Unique Set of Organisms For Each Person 11
   What Is AIDS? 12
   The CDC Definition of AIDS 13
   Exam Questions 18

Chapter 2 HIV Infection and Transmission Of The Virus 19
   Introduction 19
   How HIV Is Transmitted 20
   Risk of Transmission 20
   Who Is at Highest Risk? 23
   HIV Infection and Health Care Workers 24
   Exam Questions 25

Chapter 3 Preventing Transmission of HIV 27
   Introduction 27
   Preventing Transmission 28
   Infection Control In the Health Care Setting 30
   Health Care Workers and HIV 34
   Exam Questions 37

Chapter 4 HIV Disease In Women 39
   Introduction 39
   Epidemiology 40
   Assessment 41
   HIV Disease In Women 42
   Pregnancy 43
   Counseling and Guidelines for Safe Sex 43
   Issues Affecting Women Who Have HIV Disease 44
   Exam Questions 46

Chapter 5 HIV Disease In Infants, Children, and Adolescents 47
   Introduction 48
   Infants and Children 48
   Definition of HIV Disease in Children 50

CONTENTS — NURSING APPROACHES TO HIV/AIDS CARE

Classification of HIV Infection in Children 50
Differences Between HIV Disease In Adults and In Infants and Children 52
Clinical Manifestations of HIV Disease in Infants and Children 53
Diagnostic Evaluation and Medical Management 54
Immunizations 61
Psychosocial Issues 62
Education of Children and Parents 64
Nursing Care 64
HIV Disease in Adolescents 65
Exam Questions 68

Chapter 6 Treatment of HIV Disease 71
Introduction 71
Clinical Trials 72
Progress Against HIV 73
Virus-Receptor Inhibitors 74
Inhibitors of Reverse Transcriptase 76
Other Antiviral Agents 78
Immunotherapy 79
Combination Therapy 79
Vaccines 80
Other Therapies 81
Where To Get Treatment 81
Exam Questions 83

Chapter 7 Medical Management of Opportunistic Infections, Tumors, And AIDS Dementia Complex 85
Assessment of Persons With HIV Disease 86
Opportunistic Infections 87
Tumors 109
AIDS Dementia Complex 116
Exam Questions 118

Chapter 8 Nursing Care 121
Introduction 122
Nursing Process 122
Planning Nursing Care 123
Care Plans For Patients With HIV Disease 125
Conclusion 143
Exam Questions 144

Chapter 9 Discharge Planning, Home and Ambulatory Care 147
Introduction 148
Nursing Care Management 148
Discharge Planning 148
Home Health Care 152
Ambulatory Care 159

Conclusion 160
Exam Questions 163

Chapter 10 Psychosocial Issues 165
Introduction 165
Sources of Psychologic Stress 166
Emotional Reactions to HIV Disease 168
Psychosocial Assessment 170
Approaches to Healing 172
Nursing Attitudes 174
Psychosocial Stressors for Nurses and Their Families 175
Conclusion 176
Exam Questions 177

Chapter 11 Ethical And Legal Issues 179
Ethical Issues 180
Legal Issues 183
Estate Matters 186
Conclusion 189
Exam Questions 191

Appendix: HIV Testing In Florida 193
Glossary 197
Bibliography 201
Index
Pre-Test Key
Evaluation

PRETEST

This self-study course is designed to allow you to complete the course at your own pace. It also allows you to focus your study on areas in which you have limited knowledge of the subject.

Begin by taking the pretest. Compare your answers on the pretest with the answer key (located in the back of the book). Circle those test items that you missed. The pretest answer key indicates the course chapters that discuss the content covered in each question.

Next, read each chapter. Focus special attention on the chapters that cover the questions for which you chose incorrect answers. When you finish the course, complete the final examination.

1. Which of the following groups in the United States has the highest number of AIDS cases?

    a. Heterosexual partners of injecting drug users
    b. Injecting drug users
    c. Children of HIV-infected mothers
    d. Homosexual/bisexual men

2. HIV can be transmitted through which of the following?

    a. Urine, blood, vaginal secretions
    b. Urine, saliva, feces
    c. Blood, breast milk, saliva
    d. Blood, breast milk, semen

3. Which of the following is a known way in which HIV is transmitted?

    a. Hugging a person who has AIDS
    b. Exposure to the sweat of someone infected with HIV
    c. Donating blood
    d. Sexual intercourse with someone infected with HIV

4. How long should health care workers who have had a needle-stick injury or splash exposure to HIV be monitored?

    a. 1–2 weeks
    b. 3–6 weeks
    c. 1–2 months
    d. 3–6 months

5. Which of the following is considered an unsafe sex practice?

    a. Frottage
    b. Mutual masturbation
    c. Unprotected vaginal or anal intercourse
    d. Kissing

6. When discussing HIV infection, nurses should be prepared to educate and counsel women about all of the following except:

    a. Use of birth control methods
    b. Having sex with HIV-negative partners only
    c. Progression of HIV disease
    d. Preventing acquisition and transmission of HIV

7. Which of the following is frequently the first indicator of the presence of HIV infection in women?

   a. Pneumocystis pneumonia
   b. Mucosal candidiasis
   c. Recurrent pneumonia
   d. Pregnancy

8. Which of the following vaccines should asymptomatic HIV-infected children receive?

   a. Bacille Calmette-Guerin
   b. Oral polio
   c. Hepatitis B
   d. Measles, mumps, rubella

9. The size of the inoculum, encephalopathy, and recurrent bacterial infections are a few of the differences in HIV infection in which of the following groups?

   a. Infants and children
   b. Children and adolescents
   c. Children and adults
   d. Adolescents and adults

10. Two reasons HIV disease is becoming more prevalent in the United States are:

    a. Drug abuse and poverty
    b. Drug use and sex
    c. Lack of education and money
    d. Poverty and fear

11. What are the two most serious issues affecting transmission of HIV in children?

    a. Options besides drug abuse and pregnancy
    b. Education of children and adults
    c. Drug abuse and police protection
    d. Education and poverty

12. What two new inhibitors of reverse transcriptase are being used to treat HIV infection?

    a. Dideoxyinosine (ddI) and ribavirin
    b. Ribavirin and acyclovir
    c. Acyclovir and dideoxycytidine (ddC)
    d. Dideoxycytidine and dideoxyinosine

13. Which protozoan is the major cause of focal intracerebral lesions in patients with AIDS?

    a. *Pneumocystis carinii*
    b. *Isospora belli*
    c. *Toxoplasma gondii*
    d. *Cryptosporidium* species

14. The eye is the most common site of infection for which virus in persons with HIV disease?

    a. Herpes simplex virus
    b. Varicella-zoster virus
    c. Epstein-Barr virus
    d. Cytomegalovirus

15. Rash, nausea, vomiting, and diarrhea are side effects of which two drugs used to treat toxoplasmosis?

    a. Pyrimethamine and nicotinic acid
    b. Pyrimethamine and sulfadiazine
    c. Sulfadiazine and clindamycin
    d. Clindamycin and nicotinic acid

16. Early manifestations of AIDS dementia complex include:

    a. Disinhibition and release reflexes
    b. Global dementia and pyramidal tract signs
    c. Impaired concentration and memory loss
    d. Disorientation and psychomotor slowing

17. Having a patient with HIV infection verbalize feelings and identify personal strengths would be an appropriate outcome criterion for which sign or symptom?

    a. Anger
    b. Isolation
    c. Depression
    d. Panic

18. Alteration in bowel elimination is a nursing diagnosis for what common HIV-related problem?

    a. Anorexia
    b. Diarrhea
    c. Edema
    d. Nausea and vomiting

19. Which of the following is a sign or symptom seen in HIV infection and AIDS that would have alteration in physical regulation related to hyperthermia as a nursing diagnosis?

    a. Fever
    b. Weakness
    c. Fatigue
    d. Diarrhea

20. During the initial home evaluation, the nurse's assessment of a patient's risk factors is based on information obtained from which of the following?

    a. History and physical examination
    b. Social and dietary history
    c. Inventory of medications
    d. Mental health history

21. Lack of communication between care providers and lack of knowledge about community resources are which of the following?

    a. Benefits of discharge planning
    b. Barriers to discharge planning
    c. Barriers to case management
    d. Benefits of home care

22. What are the most common emotional reactions experienced by persons who have HIV infection?

    a. Anger, hate, fear, and denial
    b. Love, acceptance, peace, and certainty
    c. Fear, denial, isolation, and uncertainty
    d. Apathy, hate, denial, and guilt

23. Common psychologic problems that occur during the middle stage of illness in patients with AIDS include:

    a. Fear of rejection
    b. Completion of grief work
    c. Need for financial support
    d. Anticipation of death

24. What is the philosophical study of morality, moral problems, and judgments?

    a. Descriptive ethics
    b. Metaethics
    c. Ethics
    d. Normative ethics

25. The right of persons with HIV infection to have equal access to health care resources and services is an issue related to which ethical principle?

    a. Respect for persons
    b. Autonomy
    c. Fidelity
    d. Justice

INTRODUCTION

In 1981, epidemiologists in Southern California and New York realized they had a new and frightening syndrome on their hands. Unusual and overwhelming infections and tumors were developing in previously healthy young men, and after a relatively short time, most of the men died. Then the number of cases increased dramatically, and the syndrome began appearing in women, children, hemophiliacs, and drug users. Health care professionals were suddenly faced with a deadly syndrome of unknown cause, with no effective treatment and with no cure in sight (Selwyn, 1986a).

Today, nurses are on the front lines in the fight against acquired immune deficiency syndrome (AIDS). They work with patients who are infected with human immunodeficiency virus (HIV), the organism that causes AIDS. They interact with the patients' friends and families, members of the community, and health care personnel. They provide care in all areas of the health care system. They also provide education about AIDS and HIV.

Because the disease is so complex, caring for a person with HIV infection is a challenging assignment. Once HIV has weakened a patient's immune system, death due to opportunistic infections, tumors, or other disorders is almost certain. To date, approximately 65% of patients in whom AIDS has been diagnosed have died. Most patients who are seropositive for HIV have more than one medical problem at a time. They often must cope with as many as three or four problems simultaneously. In addition, patients with HIV disease may not receive the empathy and understanding normally given to persons who have life-threatening disorders. Few diseases have such a strong physical, psychologic, emotional, financial, and social impact.

Dispelling the fears associated with HIV disease is one of the primary tasks nurses must assume. Educating persons about the disease process, modes of transmission of HIV, and ways to decrease the risk of acquiring or transmitting the virus is an important part of the health care provider's role. The only way to prevent the spread of the infection is to educate the public.

The purpose of this course is to acquaint you with the spectrum of disease caused by HIV; the process by which the virus is transmitted; ways transmission can be prevented; and the special medical, nursing, psychologic, and social problems of persons infected with HIV.

CHAPTER 1

EPIDEMIOLOGY AND PATHOPHYSIOLOGY

CHAPTER OBJECTIVE

After studying this chapter, the reader will be able to describe changes in the demographics of HIV infection and how the virus affects the human body and the immune system.

LEARNING OBJECTIVES

After studying this chapter, the reader should be able to

1. Specify where in the United States AIDS was first detected and where cases occur most often now.

2. Indicate the fatality rate of AIDS in the United States.

3. Name the geographic area where HIV most likely originated.

4. Name the persons credited with isolating the virus that causes AIDS.

5. Specify which group in the United States has the number of cases of AIDS.

6. Indicate the correct functions of B cells and CD4 T cells.

7. Name the group of viruses to which HIV belongs.

8. Indicate how Kaposi's sarcoma in persons with AIDS differs from the same tumor in other persons.

9. Indicate the most frequently detected opportunistic infections in persons who have AIDS.

10. Give an example, as designated in the 1993 CDC case definition for AIDS in adults and adolescents, of an AIDS-defining infection in a person without laboratory evidence of HIV infection.

INTRODUCTION

Marie Henry and Ada Henshaw (1989) wrote that "without exception, the human immunodeficiency virus (HIV) affects every facet of an infected individual's life, and it directly impacts on all health care delivery systems. As the primary care givers, nurses are on the cutting edge of this epidemic" (p. 7). Nurses provide the demanding day-to-day care when hospitalization is necessary and follow-up assessment after the patient is discharged. They also educate patients and the patients' significant others about HIV disease and about treatment and care at home.

Finding ways to provide compassionate, effective treatment and medical care to patients with HIV disease in a health care system already strained by the increasing number of cases is a challenge. Increased knowledge about AIDS and HIV infection is one way to meet that challenge.

BEGINNING AND ENDINGS

AIDS can affect all systems of the human body. The first report of the illness that came to be known as AIDS appeared in *Morbidity and Mortality Weekly Report* (MMWR) in June 1981. *Pneumocystis carinii* pneumonia (PCP) had been diagnosed in five previously healthy, young male homosexuals in Los Angeles. Tests showed that all five had severe immunosuppression from an unknown cause (Centers for Disease Control and Prevention [CDC], 1981; Gottlieb et al., 1981). Until then, PCP usually had been seen in persons who were immunosuppressed because they had received chemotherapy for cancer or immunosuppressive drugs for organ transplantation. Because the first cases occurred among homosexual men, the disease became known as gay-related immune deficiency syndrome, or GRIDS (Follansbee et al., 1982; Mildvan et al., 1982).

In 1982, a special report ("Epidemiologic Aspects") in *The New England Journal of Medicine* summarized the efforts of scientists and medical personnel to discover the cause of this unusual complex of illnesses. By January 1982, 159 cases had been reported to the CDC, and 38% of the patients had already died. In addition, the illness was being found in two new groups: intravenous drug users and Haitians. Because male homosexuals were no longer the only group infected, the name was changed from GRIDS to acquired immune deficiency syndrome or AIDS (Castro, Hardy, & Curran, 1986; Fineberg, 1988; LaCamera, Masur, & Henderson, 1985).

By August 1983, many investigators were convinced that a transmissible agent was responsible for the immunologic defects characteristic of AIDS (Curran, 1985). However, it was not until late 1984 and early 1985 that two men in separate countries, Robert Gallo of the United States and Luc Montagnier of France, announced that a virus had been identified as the causative agent of AIDS. Further investigation showed that the virus belonged to a group known as retroviruses and was similar to several other viruses known to cause various forms of cancer (Selwyn, 1986a). The virus was called human T-cell lymphotropic virus type III (HTLV-III) by Dr. Gallo and lymphadenopathy virus (LAV) by Dr. Montagnier. In 1986, the International Nomenclature Committee named it human immunodeficiency virus, or HIV (Epstein et al., 1987).

The statistics for HIV infection and AIDS are numbing. By early 1984, more than 5,000 cases of AIDS had been reported in the United States. By March of 1989, a total of 84,000 cases had been diagnosed. The 35,328 cases reported in 1989 constituted a 9% increase over the number reported in 1988. Many of these patients were women and children (CDC, 1990a).

Since the discovery of the syndrome, AIDS has developed in the majority of persons who have tested positive for HIV. Sixty percent of AIDS cases have been reported in metropolitan areas on the east and west coasts, particularly in New York City, San Francisco, Los Angeles, and Miami (Cohen, Sande, & Volberding, 1990).

In 1990, more than 40,000 cases of AIDS, or 17.2 cases per 100,000 population, were reported. This number represented about one-fourth of all the cases reported during 1981–1990 (CDC, 1991a). Epidemiologists expect that the number of cases will continue to spiral upward. It has been estimated that 58% of all adults and 65% of all children in whom AIDS had been diagnosed by 1991 will die within 2–5 years of symptoms appearing, usually after a terrible course of debilitating disease (Office of AIDS, 1990).

The statistics for 1991 (CDC, 1991b, 1992b) revealed the following:

1. The cumulative number of AIDS cases reported in the United States since 1981 was 202,843 as of November 30, 1991.
2. 130,687 AIDS-related deaths had occurred as of November 30, 1991.
3. 43,389 newly diagnosed cases of AIDS had been reported for 1991 as of December 21, 1991.

Comparison of these data with the predictions made at a 1986 U.S. Public Health Service conference shows that the number of AIDS cases continues to increase but at a slower rate than anticipated. This lower than anticipated increase is due to many factors: a decrease in the rate of infection in male homosexuals, earlier detection of HIV infections, earlier intervention for asymptomatic HIV infection, availability of outpatient treatment, the delay in reporting of cases, and the availability of drugs effective against retroviruses. Despite these advances, however, it is anticipated that without a vaccine to prevent infection, at least 40,000 new infections will occur each year among adults and adolescents (Morgan, Curran, & Berkelman, 1990). In addition, changes in the CDC definition of AIDS became effective January 1, 1993 (see The CDC Definition of AIDS at the end of this chapter). These changes mean that more cases will be reported. It has been estimated that the new definition will account for an additional 30,000 cases each year.

As the second decade of our experience with HIV disease began, a demographic change became evident. AIDS is no longer primarily a disease of gay white males, hemophiliacs, and injecting drug users (IDUs; see chapter 2 for an explanation of this new term). From 1989 to 1990, the number of AIDS cases in heterosexual IDUs, heterosexual partners of persons infected with HIV, and infants infected at birth increased 30%. Heterosexual transmission of HIV has nearly replaced homosexual transmission in New York, New Jersey, and Florida. As heterosexual transmission has increased, so has the number of infants born with HIV infection.

In 1990, the number of reported cases per 100,000 population in the United States was higher for men, blacks, and Hispanics, and persons 30–49 years old. AIDS is the second leading cause of death in boys and men 15–45 years old, and in 1991, it was the fifth leading cause of death for girls and women in the same age group. Hispanics represent 9% of the general population, yet accounted for 16% percent of the reported cases nationwide in 1991 (Sanchez, 1992). Women accounted for more than 11% of the cases in adults and adolescents. Approximately 58% of these women were black, and 48% were IDUs. Figures 1 and 2 (p.4) provide a better picture of the demographic changes in AIDS (CDC, 1991c; "The Changing Demographics," 1991).

Although the number of cases of AIDS in the United States is high, the number of cases worldwide is stag-

Figure 1
AIDS CASES, BY YEAR OF DIAGNOSIS: UNITED STATES 1981–1990[*]

Total cases, cases among homosexual/bisexual men[†], and cases among women and heterosexual men reporting intravenous (IV) drug use

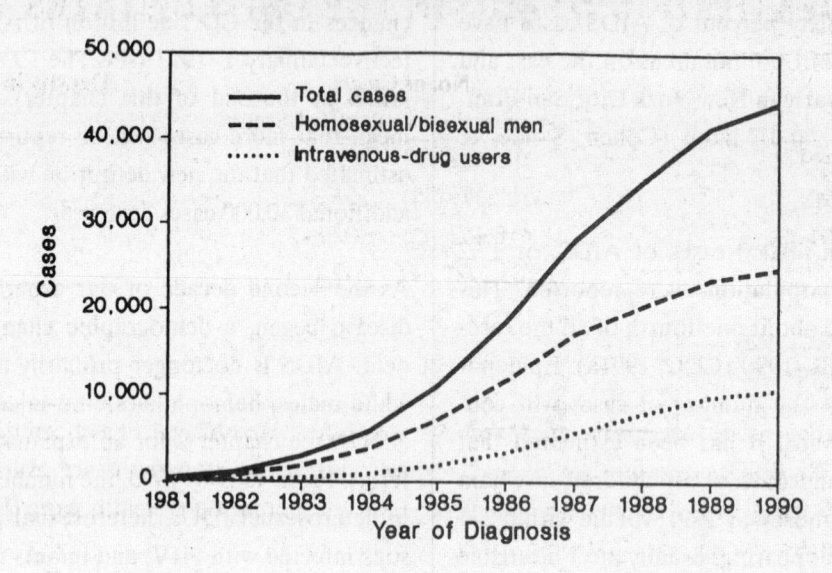

Figure 2
AIDS CASES AMONG PERSONS REPORTING HETEROSEXUAL CONTACT WITH PERSONS WITH, OR AT HIGH RISK FOR, HIV INFECTION

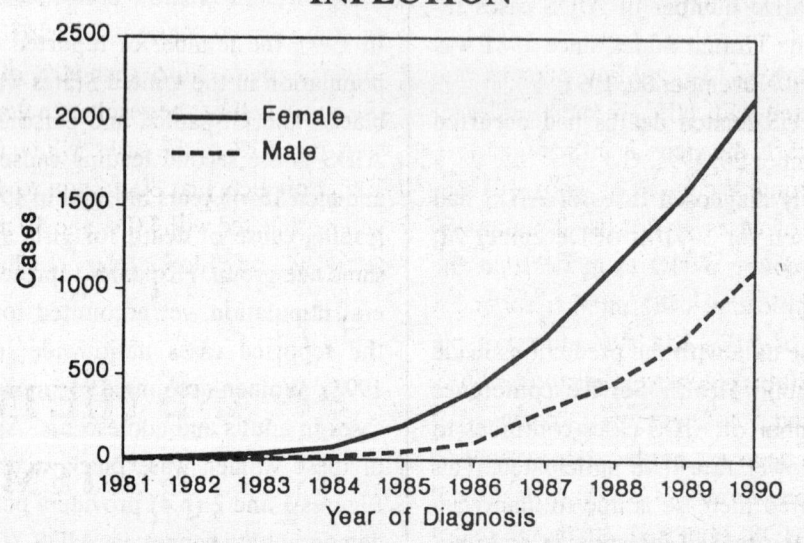

*Based on cases reported through March 1991 and adjusted for reporting delays.
†Excludes IV drug users.

Source: Centers for Disease Control, 1991c.

CHAPTER 1 —
EPIDEMIOLOGY AND PATHOPHYSIOLOGY

Table 1
CUMULATIVE NUMBER OF AIDS CASES REPORTED WORLDWIDE AND IN THE UNITED STATES AND CUMULATIVE NUMBER OF DEATHS DUE TO AIDS IN THE UNITED STATES

Date	No. of Cases Worldwide	United States	Deaths in United States
November 1989	198,165	115,158	68,441
November 1990	307,379	157,525	98,530
November 1991	418,403	202,843	130,687
1992	1,501,272*	242,146**	160,372**

*As of January 1, 1992
**As of September 1992

gering, and, in many cases, inaccurate. In March 1990, the World Health Organization (WHO) reported that 222,740 cases of AIDS had been diagnosed in 143 countries during the first months of that year. By January 1, 1992, 1.5 million cases of AIDS in 162 countries had been reported (WHO, 1992). Table 1 shows the cumulative number of AIDS cases reported in the United States, to September 1992, and worldwide to January 1, 1992 (CDC, 1991b, 1992a, 1992b; WHO, 1992).

Worldwide, as many as 10 million persons are thought to be infected with HIV. In most underdeveloped countries, early diagnosis is difficult, and reporting of the syndrome is delayed or ignored. Thus, the actual number of cases worldwide is unknown. Taking this into account, WHO estimates that the actual number is three times the number reported. Reporting of cases of AIDS has been more reliable from the United States. However, Uganda, Zaire, Zambia, Rwanda, and other equatorial Central African countries have been hit harder. It is estimated that two to three generations of Central Africans will die as a result of AIDS. Hundreds of thousands of African children have lost both parents to the illness, and many more infants and children are dying of the syndrome. Health care is inadequate, and services are nonexistent. Many African countries are able to spend only about $1 per person on health care each year. The island of Haiti has been devastated by the infection because no funds are available for education and appropriate health care (Flaskerud, 1989; Mann, 1989).

Experts are now predicting that by the year 2000, management of AIDS patients will become one of the world's largest economic and social concerns. The pandemic will have moved out of cities into rural and more remote areas. Rates of transmission in Southeast Asia and the Pacific islands will match those in Africa. More than 90% of all AIDS cases in the world will be the result of heterosexual transmission, and 50% of the cases will be in women. Finally, WHO predicts that 30 million to 40 million persons will be infected with HIV, and 10 million of those infected will be children (Nary & Challice, 1992).

HIV AND THE IMMUNE SYSTEM

What Is HIV?

HIV is a retrovirus. All retroviruses contain ribonucleic acid (RNA) as their genetic material. In addition, they have a unique viral enzyme, reverse transcriptase. The infected cell uses this enzyme to make deoxyribonucleic acid (DNA) copies of viral RNA.

HIV does not infect all types of cells. Infection is restricted to cells that bear a specific receptor for the virus. The receptor for HIV is a protein complex called CD4. The virus attaches to the receptor on the cell's surface and then penetrates or invades the cell. Penetration is required before HIV can reproduce. Helper/inducer T cells have large amounts of CD4 on their surfaces. Consequently, they are the primary target cells of HIV. Other types of cells, such as macrophages, also have CD4 on their surfaces, but the amount is much smaller. Unless otherwise specified, the term "CD4 cells" usually refers to CD4 T cells.

Once HIV penetrates the cell, it eventually directs the cell to produce more virus. The infected cell can remain in a latent state in which it makes little or no viral RNA. This latent period could be one explanation for the long incubation period during which persons infected with HIV have no signs or symptoms of HIV disease. At some point, the cells start to actively produce and release infectious virus. The virus then can infect other cells. The number of CD4 T cells decreases, and the immune system becomes impaired. Persons infected with HIV may be asymptomatic during the incubation period or may have a range of signs and symptoms as the immune response becomes weaker. Severe immunosuppression ultimately leads to opportunistic infections, tumors, or other disorders such as AIDS dementia complex.

Where Did HIV Originate?

HIV is probably the result of a new infection in humans that began appearing in Central Africa in the 1950s. Some researchers (Kanki et al., 1985; Selwyn, 1986a) theorize that a simian virus, STLV-III, somehow infected humans, perhaps through a bite by an infected monkey. The virus then mutated several times, resulting in HIV, a form that affects humans. Movement of large numbers of Africans from rural, agricultural communities to large, industrialized cities may have led to widespread dissemination of the virus.

The Normal Immune System

Normally, all components of the immune system operate in harmonious balance, protecting the body against invading organisms and foreign (nonself) antigens. Lymphocytes, important components of the system, can be divided into two distinct types: B cells and T cells (Figure 3, p.7). B cells mature in the bone marrow and can divide and differentiate into plasma cells, which produce antibodies (Selwyn, 1986a). T cells, which develop in the thymus, can be divided into four types: helper/inducer T cells (CD4 cells), suppressor T cells (CD8 cells), cytotoxic or killer T cells, and memory T cells. Although all four types play critical roles in the immune response, CD4 cells are especially important. These cells secrete chemicals, known as lymphokines, that regulate the functions of other immune cells. Lymphokines are involved in recognition of foreign antigens, proliferation of T cells, regulation of toxic and suppressor functions, and production of antibodies.

In a person with a healthy immune system (Figure 4, p.8), invading microorganisms are engulfed by phagocytic cells (neutrophils and macrophages). These cells kill the organisms (which have foreign or nonself antigens), and the remnants are delivered to CD4 cells. This activates the CD4 cells, and they begin to multiply and produce lymphokines. In addition, cytopathic T cells multiply and attack any cells in the body that have been successfully infected by the invading microorganisms. Antibodies produced as a result of B-cell activation add to the immune response. They may promote phagocytosis, neutralize toxins, or, with other components in the sera, destroy the microorganisms, or at least prevent the organisms from penetrating host cells.

One of the mysteries of HIV infection is why an infected person with a competent immune system is

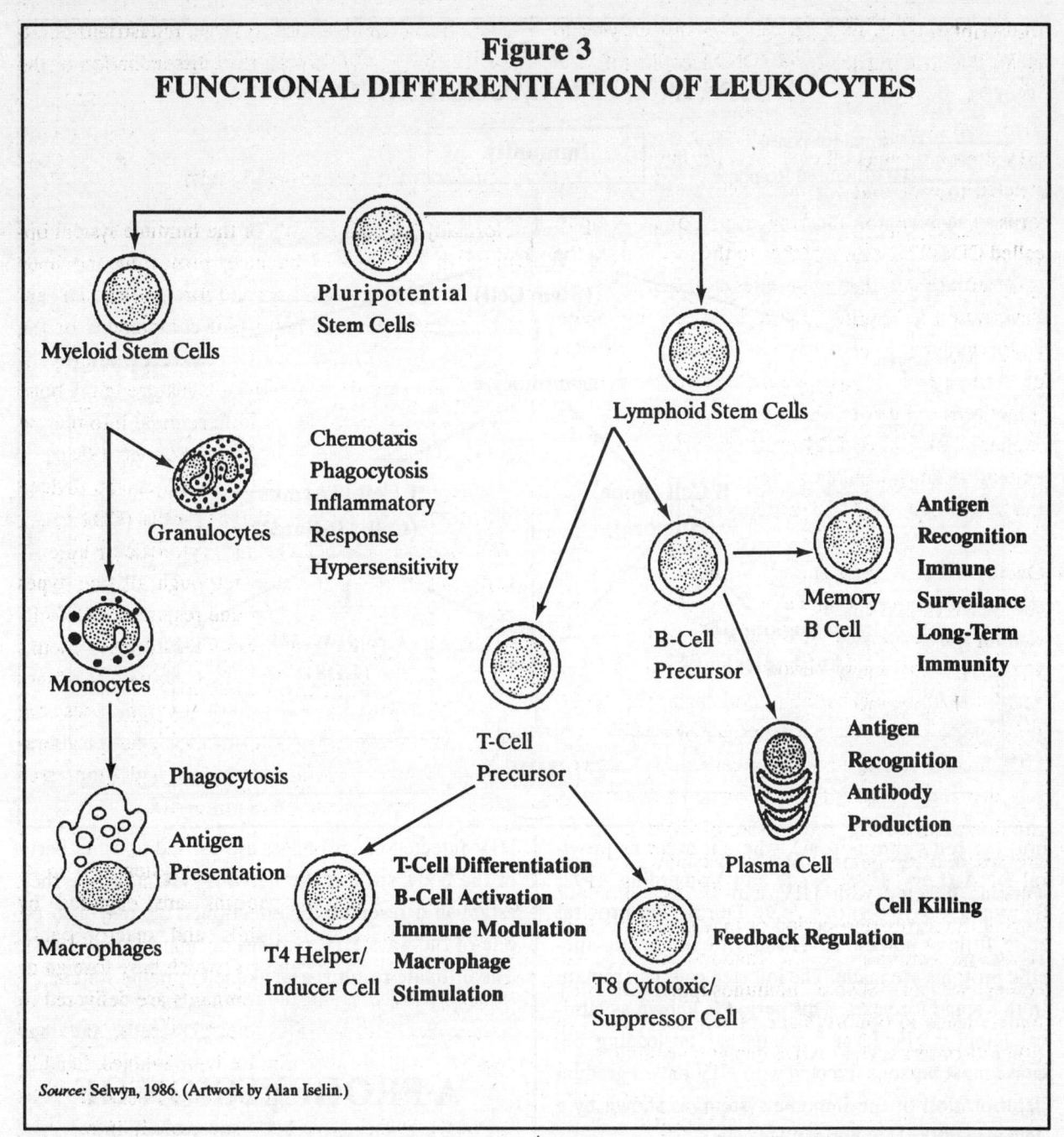

Figure 3
FUNCTIONAL DIFFERENTIATION OF LEUKOCYTES

Pluripotential Stem Cells

Myeloid Stem Cells

Lymphoid Stem Cells

Granulocytes — Chemotaxis, Phagocytosis, Inflammatory Response, Hypersensitivity

Monocytes

Macrophages — Phagocytosis, Antigen Presentation

T-Cell Precursor

B-Cell Precursor

Memory B Cell — Antigen Recognition, Immune Surveilance, Long-Term Immunity

Plasma Cell — Antigen Recognition, Antibody Production

T4 Helper/Inducer Cell — T-Cell Differentiation, B-Cell Activation, Immune Modulation, Macrophage Stimulation

T8 Cytotoxic/Suppressor Cell — Cell Killing, Feedback Regulation

Source: Selwyn, 1986. (Artwork by Alan Iselin.)

unable to control viral replication and eventually the disease. A second mystery is how the virus replicates in cells other than CD4 T cells, such as macrophages, monocytes, and neural and gastrointestinal cells (Coffin, 1990; Levy, Kaminsky, & Morrow, 1985). One possible explanation for the first mystery is that the virus mutates, which would limit the effectiveness of the immune system (Fauci, 1991).

The immune response to HIV is not the same as the response to other pathogens. As the virus circulates in the bloodstream, it comes in contact with many types of cells. When it comes in contact with a cell that has the CD4 receptor, it attaches itself to the receptor and begins to penetrate the cell. Once inside the cell, HIV releases its RNA, and the cell uses reverse transcriptase to produce double-stranded DNA copies of the viral RNA. This DNA is inserted into the nucleus of the cell and begins to be integrated

Figure 4
STEPS IN THE IMMUNE RESPONSE

— Normal Response
— HIV-Induced Response

Immunity → WBC (Stem Cell) → Monocyte, Lymphocyte, Macrophange

Lymphocyte → B Cell (Bone) (Humoral), T Cell (Thymus) (Cell-Mediated)

B Cell → Immunoglobulins (Antibodies), T Helper (CD4)

T Cell → T Helper (CD4), T Suppressor (CD8), T-Killer

HIV

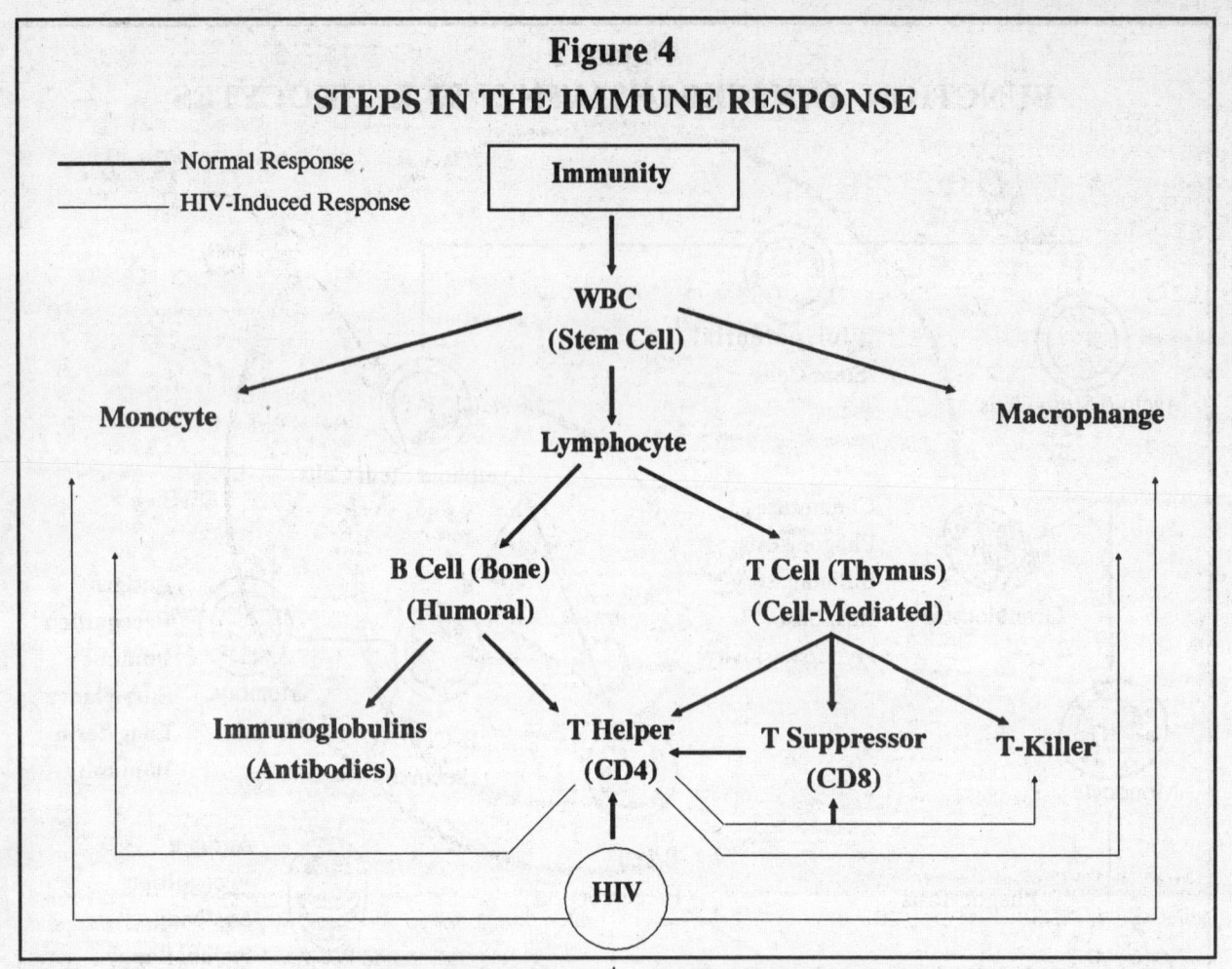

into the cell's chromosome, where it exists as proviral DNA (Levy, 1988; Sande and Volberding, 1992; Selwyn, 1986a) (Figure 5, p.9). During the proviral state, little or no viral RNA and little or no viral-specific proteins are made. The infected cells can remain in this stage for years. This period is known as clinical latency. The term is somewhat misleading because most persons infected with HIV have a gradual deterioration of the immune system, as shown by a decrease in the number of CD4 cells.

Infected cells can also enter an active production phase. The proviral DNA is used to produce viral RNA and proteins that form new copies of HIV. These virus particles or virions are released from the nucleus of the cell into the cytoplasm. They then bud from the cell surface into the bloodstream to begin the process again. Infected cells can also spread the virus by fusing with uninfected cells. In addition, HIV-infected macrophages are carried to other parts of the body, such as the nervous system, where they establish a reservoir of infection. This may also be one of the ways HIV remains dormant (Levy, 1988). The ultimate result is a weakened immune system.

A PROGRESSION OF DISEASE

HIV disease is now recognized as a chronic illness (Figure 6, p.10) with a long period of clinical latency. The disease begins with HIV infection. AIDS occurs later in the course of the disease and is diagnosed

Figure 5
HIV REPLICATION CYCLE

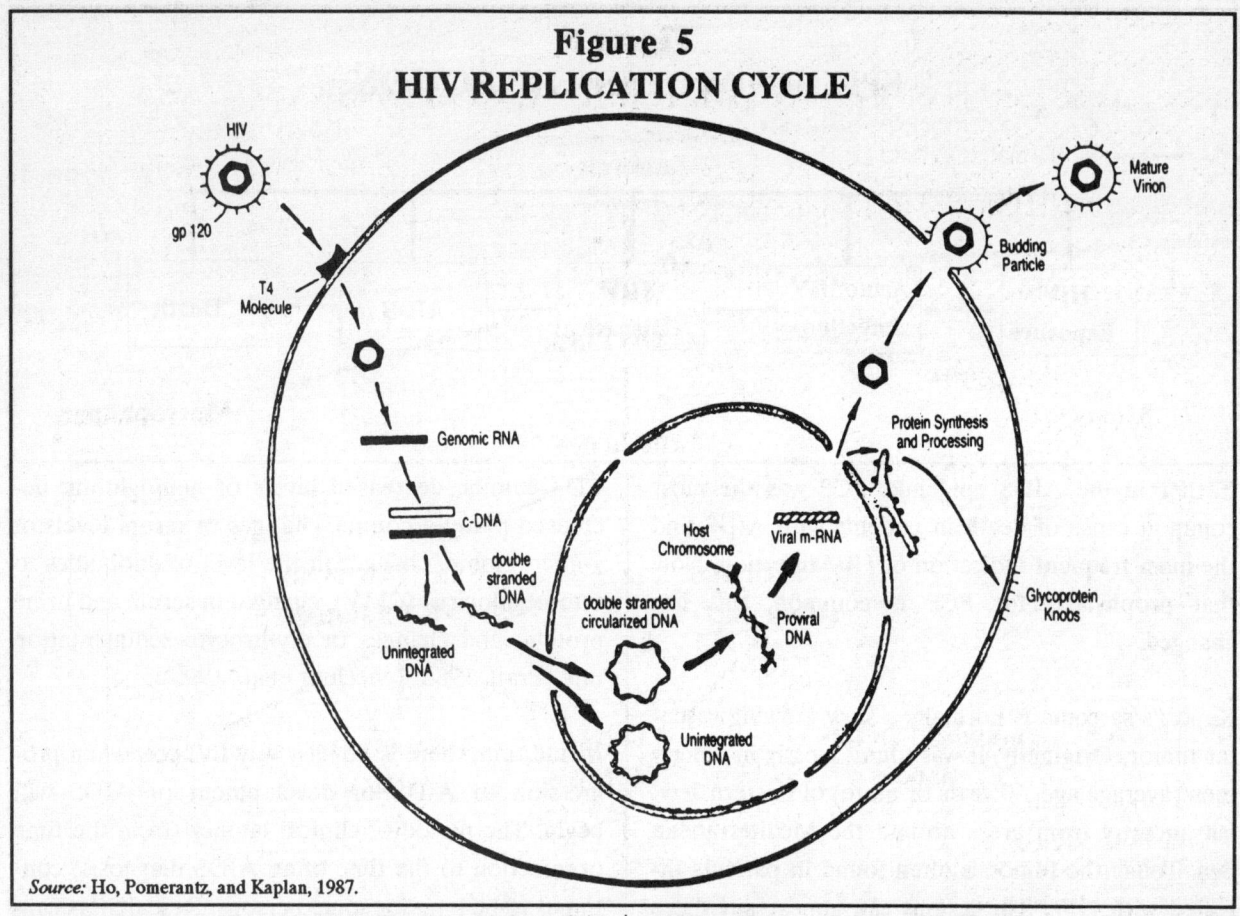

Source: Ho, Pomerantz, and Kaplan, 1987.

after the HIV-infected person has an "AIDS-defining" illness.

Most persons infected with HIV initially have an acute flulike illness. This is called acute HIV syndrome. The signs and symptoms are similar to those of other viral illnesses, including mononucleosis. They may include lymphadenopathy, fever, rash, sore throat, fatigue, myalgias, gastrointestinal problems, and diarrhea (Cohen et al., 1990; Pantaleo, Graziosi, & Fauci, 1993).

After resolution of the initial infection, a person may be asymptomatic for months to years. The average length of the clinical latency is 10 years (Pantaleo et al., 1993). Indications that the disease is progressing may include persistent generalized lymphadenopathy, a decrease in the number of CD4 cells, weight loss, or loss of an immune response to skin tests for such things as mumps virus, *Candida*, and tetanus toxoid. As the illness progresses, the number of CD4 cells continues to decrease. When the count drops to 500 cells/mm^3, some infected persons may experience fatigue, lethargy, fever, night sweats, rashes or skin lesions, oral candidiasis (thrush), or oral hairy leukoplakia. Changes may also occur in the complete blood cell count (CBC). These may include leukopenia, anemia, and thrombocytopenia. This phase, referred to in the past as AIDS-related complex (ARC), is now called symptomatic HIV disease.

As the number of CD4 cells continues to decrease, the person infected with HIV becomes susceptible to a variety of illnesses. The CDC has designated certain illnesses as AIDS-defining criteria. *Pneumocystis carinii* pneumonia (PCP) and Kaposi's sarcoma are examples of such illnesses. When the CD4 count decreases to 200 cells/mm^3, the risk of acquiring such illnesses increases. (For further information on AIDS-defining criteria, see the section titled The CDC Definition of AIDS at the end of this chapter.)

Figure 6
SPECTRUM OF HIV INFECTION

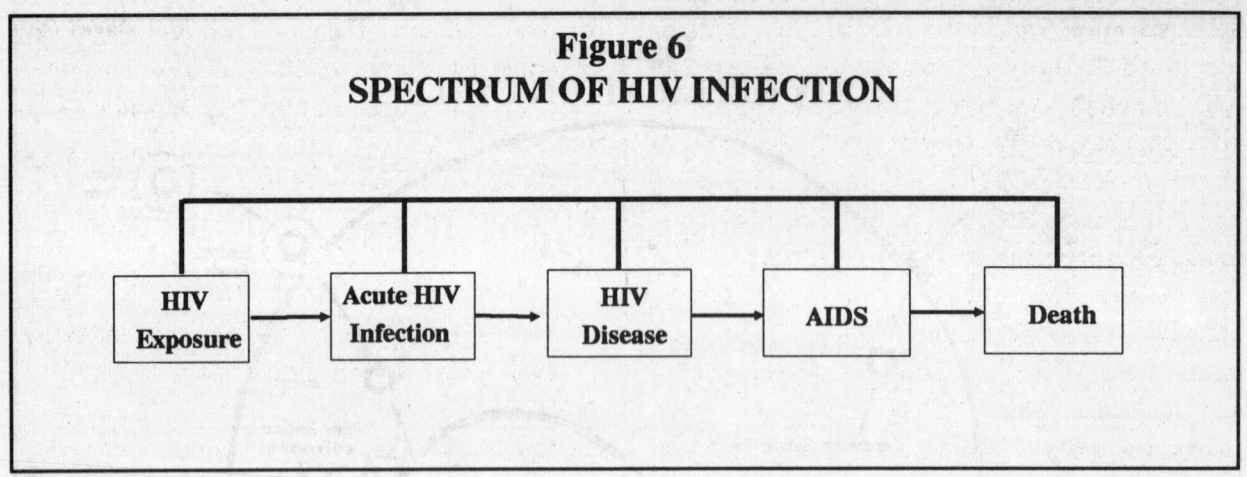

HIV Exposure → Acute HIV Infection → HIV Disease → AIDS → Death

Earlier in the AIDS epidemic, PCP was the most common cause of death in patients with AIDS and the most frequent indication of HIV infection. Now that prophylaxis for PCP is common, this has changed.

Kaposi's sarcoma is normally a slow-growing vascular tumor. Originally, it was found mostly in elderly men (average age, 60 years or more) of Eastern Jewish ancestry from areas around the Mediterranean Sea. Today the tumor is often found in patients infected with HIV. The lesions can appear anywhere on the skin and mucous membranes, but they occur most often on the lower extremities. In persons with HIV infection, the tumors grow rapidly and can affect all systems of the body, including the lungs and gastrointestinal tract.

As advances in medicine and knowledge about HIV disease are made, illnesses that used to be fatal can be prevented. However, until the primary viral infection can be treated, the immune system will continue to weaken, and eventually an illness will end in death.

Who Will Go on to Have AIDS?

Progression from asymptomatic HIV disease to AIDS does not follow a single, clear-cut path. However, certain conditions indicate that the disease is progressing. These include weight loss, fevers, night sweats, oral hairy leukoplakia, thrush, decreasing CD4 counts, decreased levels of hemoglobin, decreased platelet counts, changes in serum levels of $_2$-microglobin, changes in the level of antibodies to cytomegalovirus (CMV), changes in serum and urine protein, and changes in erythrocyte sedimentation rate (Pratt, 1986; Schechter et al., 1990).

In addition, there is no easy way to know when progression to AIDS or development of AIDS will begin. The period of clinical latency (from the time of infection to the time of an AIDS diagnosis) continues to be long for some persons. Researchers cannot pinpoint why AIDS develops in persons infected with HIV. Consequently, some investigators think that one or more factors may be working with the virus to trigger the onset of AIDS. Others think that development of AIDS does not require the presence of HIV (DeLoughry, 1991). Instead, they postulate, conditions, such as drug abuse and malnutrition, suppress the immune system and lead to AIDS.

In a recent article, Schechter et al. (1990) stated that some of the factors responsible for a more rapid progression to AIDS may be present in the host before or shortly after the HIV infection is established. These include genetics, high initial viral load, and biological properties of HIV variants. The authors also indicated that the occurrence of signs and symptoms near the time of seroconversion is associated with an increased rate of progression to AIDS.

Some scientists hypothesize that HIV has a minor role in AIDS. They think that the patients in whom AIDS develops have factors in common other than HIV. They suggest that the combined impact of HIV and other viruses such as Epstein-Barr virus (EBV), hepatitis B virus (HBV), or herpesviruses should be examined. They think that the role of other factors that suppress the immune system should also be evaluated. These include malnutrition, blood transfusions, cocaine use, overuse of antibiotics, syphilis, and gonorrhea. Finally, a segment of this group thinks that everyone is infected with HIV and that the virus is activated and AIDS develops only in those who have the foregoing factors. All these ideas are still being discussed. The role of these cofactors is currently being studied (DeLoughry, 1991).

As a final note on this confusing issue, Rutherford and Lifson (Clark, 1990) stated at the 6th International Conference on AIDS that some persons infected with HIV may never have signs and symptoms of AIDS. They also indicated that the risk of AIDS developing increases with the length of time a person is infected, but, currently, the disease can no longer be called invariably fatal.

Staging of HIV Infection

The spectrum of HIV infection is best understood when it is organized into a system that indicates how the disease progresses. The first staging system was developed by the military and incorporated clinical and immunologic parameters. It was used to determine which persons infected with HIV should remain in the military and which would be discharged (Redfield, Wright, & Fremont, 1986). In 1986, the CDC staging system (Table 2, p.12; CDC, 1986b) was published. This system is based on clinical findings.

Nursing has also developed staging systems. Sedaka and O'Reilly (1986) developed Stages of Deterioration: AIDS/ARC Intervention to help the Visiting Nurses Association in Los Angeles design a flexible care delivery model that includes appropriate and compassionate care. The model has four stages (see following). Each stage is defined by signs and symptoms of illness and psychologic impact, and each includes interventions needed.

Stage 1: Prediagnosis to diagnosis of AIDS or ARC

Stage 2: First opportunistic infection and/or obvious multisystem involvement—AIDS/ARC

Stage 3: Repetitive opportunistic infections/multisystem failures

Stage 4: Actively dying

Schietinger (1986) developed a staging system to help with the treatment of persons infected with HIV. Her system is linear and recognizes that HIV infection is a continuum rather than one illness that resolves.

A UNIQUE SET OF PATHOGENS FOR EACH PERSON

HIV disease must be viewed as a continuum: It begins with the mild signs and symptoms of the initial infection with HIV, progresses through the generalized lymphadenopathy syndrome, and finally ends in AIDS. However, not all patients follow a "normal" progression. Each person infected with HIV has a unique disease process. The development of opportunistic infections, tumors, and other illnesses and the additional ramifications of HIV disease are different for each patient.

The immunosuppression caused by HIV can lead to activation or reactivation of latent infections. Since

Table 2
STAGING SYSTEM

Group	Characteristics
Group I	Acute infection
Group II	Asymptomatic infection
Group III	Persistent generalized lymphadenopathy
Group IV	Other diseases
Subgroup A	Constitutional diseases
Subgroup B	Neurologic diseases
Subgroup C	Secondary infectious diseases
Category C-1	Specified secondary infectious diseases listed in the CDC surveillance definition of AIDS
Category C-2	Other specified secondary infectious diseases
Subgroup D	Secondary cancers
Subgroup E	Other conditions

Source: Centers for Disease Control, 1986b.

pathogens vary from region to region, certain infections may be more common in certain regions. Thus, the infections that occur in a person with HIV disease are determined by where the person has traveled and lived. This probably accounts for the variations among patients from different parts of the country, with different life-styles and different health histories.

WHAT IS AIDS?

In 1986, AIDS was defined as a group of diseases or tumors that indicated an underlying cellular immunodeficiency in a person who did not have an underlying immune deficiency state, who had not received medications that could cause immunosuppression, and who did not have a malignant neoplasm (Abrams, Dilley, Maxey, & Volberding, 1986). The syndrome of AIDS is diagnosed according to criteria established by the CDC in 1987. Persons with AIDS are those who (1) have or are suspected of having HIV infection and (2) meet the CDC criteria for the diagnosis of AIDS.

However, the CDC has recently made changes in the surveillance definition. As of January 1, 1993, a person is classified as having AIDS if he or she has a CD4 count of less than 200 cells/mm^3 or the development of opportunistic infections, including pulmonary tuberculosis and recurrent pneumonias, or cervical neoplasia or tumors (CDC, 1992c).

THE CDC DEFINITION OF AIDS

The CDC has developed criteria for the diagnosis and classification of HIV disease (CDC, 1987d). Figure 7 (p.14) is a flow diagram that can be used to determine if a patient has AIDS (CDC, 1992c).

The classification system for adults and adolescents is a categorization of conditions associated with HIV infection. The 1987 classification system was based on diseases only. The revised classification system includes patients whose CD4 count is less than 200 cells/mm^3, which indicates severe immunodeficiency. Tuberculosis, recurrent bacterial pneumonias, and cervical neoplasia are included as indicator conditions. This means that anyone whose CD4 count is less than 200 cells/mm^3 or who has an AIDS-related disease listed in the surveillance definition will have a diagnosis of AIDS.

The new surveillance case definition is an attempt to include patients who have severe defects in their immune system but no opportunistic infections or tumors. It is hoped that the new definition will comprehensively represent both men and women who have severe immunodeficiency. It will also be consistent with standards of medical care, simplify the reporting process, better categorize HIV-related illnesses, and lead to a more accurate indication of the number of persons with severe HIV-related immunosuppression (Howe, 1991b).

The following gives the CDC 1993 case definition for AIDS in adults and adolescents (CDC, 1992c):

For national reporting, a case of AIDS is defined as an illness characterized by one or more of the following indicator conditions, depending on the status of laboratory evidence of HIV infection, as shown in the following.

I. Patients Without Laboratory Evidence of HIV Infection: If laboratory tests for HIV were not done or the results were inconclusive, and if the patient had no other cause of immunodeficiency (see Section I.A), then any disease listed in Section I indicates AIDS if it was diagnosed by a definitive method.

    A. Causes of immunodeficiency that disqualify diseases as indicators of AIDS in the absence of laboratory evidence of HIV infection

        1. High-dose or long-term systemic corticosteroid therapy or other immunosuppressive/cytotoxic therapy 3 months or less before the onset of the indicator disease

        2. Any of the following diseases diagnosed 3 months or less before diagnosis of the indicator disease:

            a. Hodgkin's disease

            b. Non-Hodgkin's lymphoma (other than primary brain lymphoma)

            c. Lymphocytic leukemia

            d. Multiple myeloma or any other cancer of lymphoreticular or histiocytic tissue, or angioimmunoblastic lymphadenopathy

        3. A genetic (congenital) immunodeficiency syndrome or an acquired immunodeficiency syndrome atypical of HIV infection, such as one involving hypogammaglobulinemia

    B. Indicator diseases diagnosed definitively

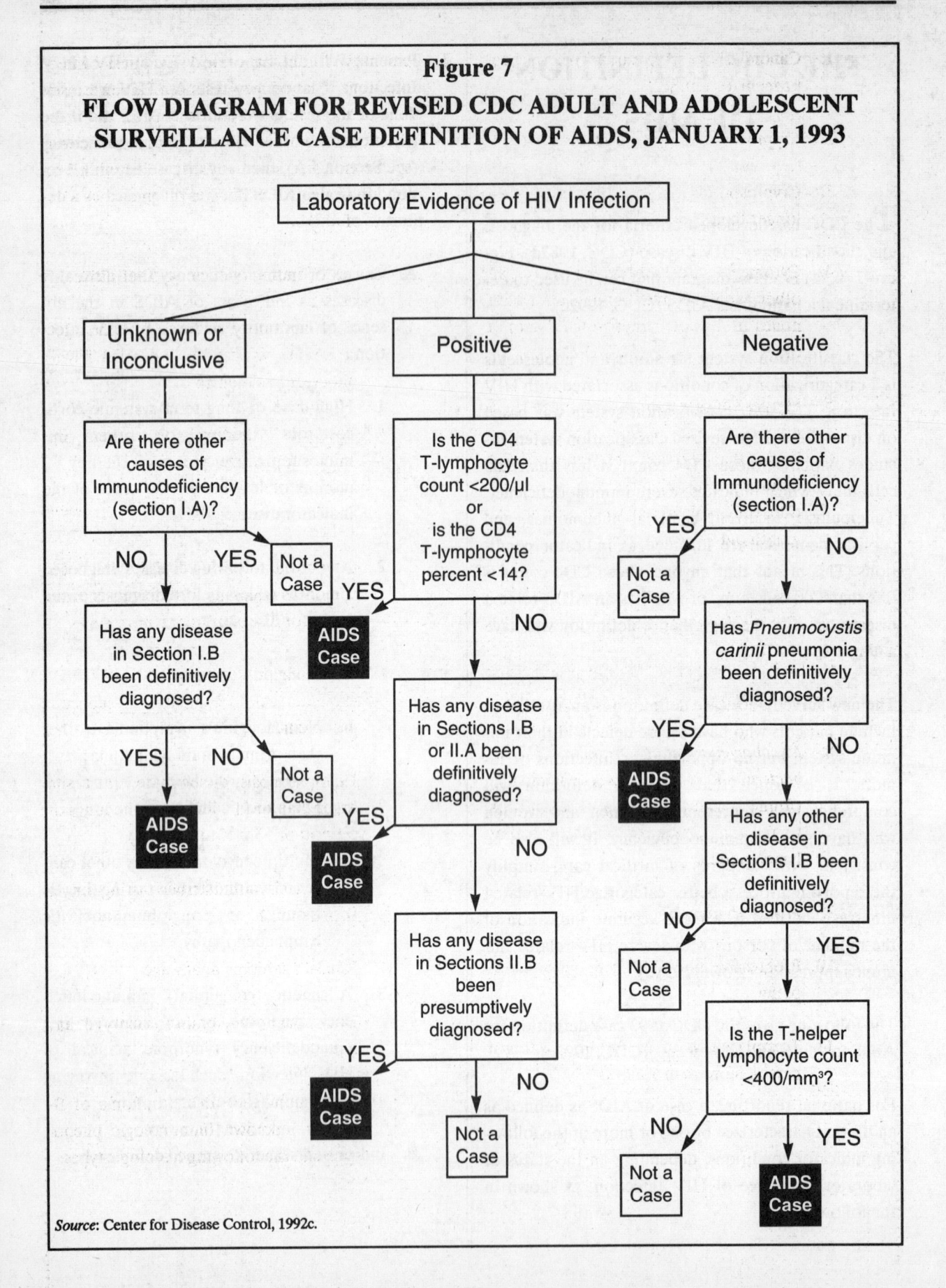

Figure 7
FLOW DIAGRAM FOR REVISED CDC ADULT AND ADOLESCENT SURVEILLANCE CASE DEFINITION OF AIDS, JANUARY 1, 1993

Source: Center for Disease Control, 1992c.

CHAPTER 1 —
EPIDEMIOLOGY AND PATHOPHYSIOLOGY

1. Candidiasis of the esophagus, trachea, bronchi, or lungs

2. Cryptococcosis, extrapulmonary

3. Cryptosporidiosis, with diarrhea lasting longer than 1 month

4. Cytomegalovirus disease of an organ other than the liver, spleen, or lymph nodes in a patient more than 1 month old

5. Herpes simplex viral infection causing a mucocutaneous ulcer that persists longer than 1 month; bronchitis, pneumonitis, or esophagitis, for any duration, which affects a patient more than 1 month old

6. Kaposi's sarcoma affecting a patient less than 60 years old

7. Lymphoma of the brain (primary) affecting a person less than 60 years old

8. *Mycobacterium avium* complex or *Mycobacterium kansasii* disease, disseminated (found at a site other than or in addition to the lungs, skin, or cervical or hilar lymph nodes)

9. *Pneumocystis carinii* pneumonia

10. Progressive multifocal leukoencephalopathy

11. Toxoplasmosis of the brain affecting a person more than 1 month old

II. Persons with Laboratory Evidence of HIV Infection: Regardless of the presence of other causes of immunodeficiency (Section I.A), in the presence of laboratory evidence for HIV infection, any disease listed in the preceding Section I.B or the following Sections II.A or II.B indicates a diagnosis of AIDS.

A. Indicator conditions diagnosed definitively

1. CD4 T-lymphocyte count less than 200 cells/mm^3, or percentage of CD4 T lymphocytes less than 14

2. Recurrent pneumonia, more than one episode in a 1-year period

3. Cervical cancer, invasive

4. Coccidioidomycosis, disseminated (at a site other than or in addition to the lungs or cervical or hilar lymph nodes)

5. HIV encephalopathy (also called HIV dementia, AIDS dementia, or subacute encephalitis due to HIV)

6. Histoplasmosis, disseminated (at a site other than or in addition to the lungs or cervical or hilar lymph nodes)

7. Isosporiasis with diarrhea lasting longer than 1 month

8. Kaposi's sarcoma at any age

9. Lymphoma of the brain (primary) at any age

10. Other non-Hodgkin's lymphoma of B-cell or unknown immunologic phenotype and the following histologic types:

a. Small noncleaved lymphoma (either Burkitt's or non-Burkitt's type)

b. Immunoblastic sarcoma (equivalent to any of the following, although not necessarily all in combination: immunoblastic lymphoma, large-cell lymphoma, diffuse undifferentiated lymphoma, or high-grade lymphoma)

Note: The CDC does not include lymphomas in this category if they are of T-cell immunologic phenotype or if their histologic type is not described or is described as lymphocytic, lymphoblastic, small-cleaved, or plasmacytoid lymphocytic.

11. Any mycobacterial disease caused by mycobacteria other than *Mycobacterium tuberculosis,* disseminated (at a site other than or in addition to the lungs, skin, or cervical or hilar lymph nodes)

12. Disease caused by *M. tuberculosis,* pulmonary or extrapulmonary

13. *Salmonella* (nontyphoid) septicemia, recurrent

14. HIV wasting syndrome ("slim disease," emaciation)

B. Indicator diseases diagnosed presumptively

Note: Given the seriousness of diseases indicative of AIDS, it is generally important to diagnose them definitively, especially when therapy that would be used may have serious side effects or when definitive diagnosis is needed for eligibility for antiretroviral therapy. Nonetheless, in some situations, a patient's condition will not permit the performance of definitive tests. In other situations, accepted clinical practice may be to make a presumptive diagnosis based on the presence of characteristic clinical and laboratory abnormalities.

1. Recurrent pneumonia, more than one episode in a 1-year period

2. Candidiasis of the esophagus

3. Cytomegalovirus retinitis with loss of vision

4. Kaposi's sarcoma

5. *M. tuberculosis*, pulmonary

6. Mycobacterial disease (acid-fast bacilli with species not identified on culture), disseminated (involving at least one site other than or in addition to the lungs, skin, or cervical or hilar lymph nodes)

7. *Pneumocystis carinii* pneumonia

8. Toxoplasmosis of the brain affecting a person more than 1 month old

III. Persons with Laboratory Evidence Against HIV Infection: With laboratory test results negative for HIV infection, a diagnosis of AIDS for surveillance purposes is ruled out unless

A. All other causes of immunodeficiency listed in Section I.A are excluded; AND

B. The patient has had either

1. *Pneumocystis carinii* pneumonia diagnosed by a definitive method; OR

2. a. Any of the other diseases that are indicative of AIDS listed in Section I.B diagnosed by a definitive method; AND

b. A T-helper/inducer (CD4) lymphocyte count less than 400 cells/mm^3

The next chapter examines risk behaviors in transmission of HIV and ways to control and prevent transmission.

EXAM QUESTIONS

Chapter 1

Questions 1 - 7

1. Which of the following is an example of an AIDS-defining infection in a person without laboratory evidence of HIV infection?

   a. *Candida* esophagitis
   b. Pulmonary *Mycobacterium tuberculosis* infection
   c. Recurrent pneumonia
   d. Disseminated histoplasmosis

2. Which cells develop in the thymus and become the mastermind of the immune system?

   a. Red cells
   b. Platelets
   c. T cells
   d. B cells

3. Which cells develop in the bone marrow and are responsible for production of antibodies to foreign antigens?

   a. Red cells
   b. Mast cells
   c. B cells
   d. T cells

4. Which of the following groups in the United States has the highest number of AIDS cases?

   a. Homosexual/bisexual men
   b. Injecting drug users
   c. Children of HIV-infected mothers
   d. Heterosexual partners of injecting drug users

5. What kind of virus is HIV?

   a. Herpesvirus
   b. Papovavirus
   c. Simian virus
   d. Retrovirus

6. The difference between Kaposi's sarcoma in a person who is seronegative for HIV and Kaposi's sarcoma in a patient with AIDS is that in a patient with AIDS the tumor is found in what part of the body?

   a. Throughout the body
   b. On the mucous membranes in the mouth only
   c. In the brain only
   d. In the eyes only

7. What is the most frequently detected opportunistic infection in patients with AIDS?

   a. *Mycobacterium tuberculosis* infection
   b. Toxoplasmosis
   c. Cryptococcosis
   d. *Pneumocystis carinii* pneumonia

CHAPTER 2

HIV INFECTION AND TRANSMISSION OF THE VIRUS

CHAPTER OBJECTIVE

After studying this chapter, the reader will be able to describe how HIV is transmitted and indicate which populations are at risk for HIV infection.

LEARNING OBJECTIVES

After studying this chapter, the reader should be able to

1. Specify three known ways in which HIV is transmitted.

2. Specify the behavior that places IDUs at an increased risk for HIV infection.

3. Indicate the year in which a nationwide program for screening donated blood was started in the United States.

4. Describe behaviors that increase the risk of becoming infected with HIV.

5. Specify the risk of HIV infection for health care workers exposed to HIV by needle-stick injuries or by contact with the body fluids of an infected person.

INTRODUCTION

HIV is an equal-opportunity organism. Under the right circumstances, anyone can become infected with it, regardless of sex, age, race, sexual preference, social stature, or address. However, certain behaviors, practices, and health situations increase the risk of exposure to the virus. These include sex with multiple partners, sex with a person who is at risk for HIV or is bisexual, use of injectable drugs, and treatment with blood or blood products (blood transfusions).

HOW HIV IS TRANSMITTED

Theoretically, HIV could be found in any body fluid that contains lymphocytes. Thus, hypothetically, exposure to any fluid containing HIV could pose a risk of transmission. Other modes of transmission also have been suggested. However, the results of many studies indicate that HIV can be transmitted only by direct transfer of body fluids (Lifson, 1988). This means that the virus is transmitted only by direct blood-to-blood contact, through sexual intercourse, or from an HIV-infected woman to her fetus or infant.

HIV is a blood-borne pathogen similar to hepatitis B virus (HBV). Two components are necessary for the transmission of blood-borne viruses:

1. The presence of the virus in sufficient quantity.

2. A means of entry into the bloodstream that permits the virus to infect cells.

For HIV infection to become established, the virus must be delivered to a susceptible host. Thus far, HIV has been isolated from samples of blood, plasma, lymph node tissue, bone marrow cells, cerebrospinal fluid, brain tissue, semen, cervical and vaginal secretions, amniotic fluid, breast milk, lung tissue, pleural fluid, peritoneal fluid, synovial fluid, saliva, and tears. However, only those body fluids that contain blood or those that potentially could contain blood have been implicated in transmission of the virus. In addition, HIV is not the only blood-borne pathogen capable of causing infection. For example, hepatitis B can be spread by contact with blood or body fluids of persons who are infected with HBV. For this reason, all blood and body fluids should be considered infective.

Studies have shown that the following are the only ways HIV can be transmitted:

1. Sexual intercourse with an HIV-infected person, during which an uninfected person is exposed to semen, cervical or vaginal secretions, or blood that contains the virus.

2. Exposure to infected blood or blood products through transfusions or through sharing of needles or other equipment that allows blood to pass from one person to another.

3. Passage of the virus from an HIV-infected mother to her infant in utero, during childbirth, or through breast milk.

RISK OF TRANSMISSION

The routine risk of infection with HIV is similar to the risk that pregnancy will occur when birth control is not used during heterosexual vaginal intercourse. For pregnancy to occur, an ovum must be exposed to sperm. It may occur after the first exposure, 1000 exposures, or any number of exposures. Likewise, HIV infection may occur after the first exposure to the virus, 1000 exposures, or any number of exposures.

Yarandi and Simpson (1991) have proposed a logistic regression model for determining the odds that a person will become infected with HIV. Using this model, they found that for a person who lived in north-central Florida and had unprotected sex (no condoms) with 20 short-term sexual partners over a 10-year period, the probability of becoming infected would be as follows:

- 4.8% if the person (male or female) had no other risk factors for HIV (i.e., was not homosexual or bisexual, did not use drugs, and so forth).

- 17.9% if the person were male and engaged in anal intercourse 50% of the time.

- 48.5% if the person were male and engaged in anal intercourse 100% of the time.

- 99.5% if the person were male and had engaged in anal intercourse 100% of the time, had both syphilis and hepatitis, and used injectable and noninjectable drugs.

- 0.66% if the person were female and had no other risk factors.

- 5.2% if the person were female and used injectable and noninjectable drugs.

The absolute risk of acquiring HIV infection during sexual intercourse is unknown. The risk depends on two variables. The first is the number of sexual contacts with an infected partner. The second is the possibility that HIV will be transmitted during sexual contact with an infected partner. This includes issues such as use of a condom or spermicide and the type of sexual activities engaged in by the participants.

The number of sexual contacts with an infected partner depends on the number of partners, the number of sexual contacts with each partner, and the prevalence of infection in the sexual contacts. The risk of transmission depends on the anatomic area that is exposed and the type of body fluid to which the uninfected partner is exposed. HIV infection is more likely to occur if one or more of the participants has some other sexually transmitted disease.

Sexual Transmission

Sexual transmission of HIV occurs in homosexuals, bisexuals, and heterosexuals. At first, most cases of AIDS were among homosexual men. In 1991, however, heterosexual transmission of HIV began to surpass homosexual transmission. In addition, one study (Padian, Shiboski, & Jewell, 1991) found that the ratio for transmission of HIV from infected males to female partners was 20:1. This means that the odds of male-to-female transmission would be much greater than the odds of female-to-male transmission. An analysis of the expected trends of AIDS cases in the United States predicted that the infection rate among heterosexuals who do not use drugs will increase. By 1995, with no changes in sexual behavior, the number of cases of AIDS in heterosexuals will be double the 10,279 cases reported through July 1991 (Allen & Setlow, 1991).

Padian et al. (1991) found that bleeding during intercourse increases the possibility of HIV transmission. Sexual activities that may cause trauma, such as receptive anal intercourse and vaginal intercourse, are thought to enhance transmission of HIV. They allow the virus to enter the bloodstream directly through damaged blood vessels or tears in the mucosa. It is important to recognize that anal intercourse is not restricted to homosexual males. In some cultures, anal intercourse is used as a means of birth control, as a way to preserve virginity, and during menstruation.

A study in male and female Africans found that HIV was spread more rapidly when other sexually transmitted diseases were present. The most common of these diseases was chancroid, which is an open draining sore (Clumeck, Van de Perre, Carael, Rouvroy, & Nzaramba, 1985). Any type of open sore increases the chance of HIV transmission.

Other persons at higher risk for HIV infection are those who have multiple sexual partners (Pratt, 1986). Many women who have more than one sexual partner use birth control pills to prevent pregnancy. However, this practice may place them at increased risk for HIV, because oral contraceptives may cause cervical erosion. An eroded cervix provides an excellent port of entry for HIV as well as for other disease-causing organisms. Intrauterine devices may also increase the risk of acquiring HIV.

Use of Injectable Drugs

Ongoing epidemiologic studies have shown that some drug users do not inject drugs directly into veins. Drugs such as cocaine and heroin may be injected under the skin (skin popping), and body-building steroids are injected into muscles. As a result, the term "injecting drug user" (IDU) is used now in place of "IV drug abuser."

Use of injectable drugs provides another major route for the spread of HIV via the blood. Sharing needles and drug equipment without cleaning them increases the risk of transmission (Howe, 1991a). HIV is transmitted directly, via the contaminated needle, from the blood of an HIV-infected IDU to the next person who uses the needle. For transmission to occur, the infected blood must be introduced directly into the bloodstream, into a vascular area under the skin, or into the muscle. Contaminated blood that falls onto intact skin or on food is not sufficient to cause subsequent infection.

In the United States, HIV infection among IDUs is on the rise, especially on the East Coast. The infection is strongly associated with the number of persons with whom needles are shared, use of "shooting galleries," and belonging to a nonwhite race (Wofsy, 1988). (Shooting galleries are houses or buildings where persons gather to do drugs. They sit together in a room and share drugs and drug equipment.)

Substance abuse means more than simply taking drugs or drinking alcohol. Both alcohol and street drugs reduce inhibitions and impair judgment. As a result, users may take part in sexual acts that they normally would avoid. Many times, the user does not remember taking part in these acts. Crack cocaine has been associated with an increase in sexual activity and promiscuity (Allen & Setlow, 1991).

Sex and drugs have created an especially fatal triangle: use of crack, resurgence of syphilis, and further spread of HIV. Crack users lose their sense of responsiblity to others (Stern, 1990), and use of the drug often leads to indiscriminate sexual activity, which increases the odds of exposure to HIV and the risk of transmission (Bernstein, MacKenzie, Oleske, & Pizzo, 1989).

To support their drug habits, many IDUs (male and female) prostitute themselves and/or their partners. In addition, for many, their families consist of needle-sharing friends and girlfriends or boyfriends, as well as relatives. Within this "family" setting, it is a matter of trust that anyone who is infected with HIV (or HBV) will use the needle last. In reality, infected IDUs do not want anyone else to know that they are infected. Consequently, they do not always use the needle last.

Blood and Blood Products

Blood transfusions have also been a means of spreading HIV. In 1982, the first cases of AIDS in hemophiliacs and transfusion recipients were reported (Eyster et al., 1985). This led to the discovery that AIDS was a disease that could be transmitted by blood. This, in turn, resulted in an all-out effort to protect the safety of the nation's banked blood supply. By 1985, screening of all donated blood for possible exposure to HIV was introduced by blood collection agencies throughout the United States and in many foreign countries. Screening procedures include tests for antibodies to HIV and interviews and questions about risk behaviors that indicate the donor might be infected with HIV.

Although all donated blood is screened now before it is added to a blood bank's inventory, the screening system is not foolproof. Antibodies to HIV do not develop immediately. In most persons, they are detectable by 6 weeks after infection. If a person is tested for HIV antibodies before the antibodies develop, the result will be falsely negative (Krim, 1986). The time between infection and the development of antibodies is called "the window."

Maternal Transmission

Infants can acquire HIV infection in utero, during birth, or from their mothers' breast milk. Approximately 30% of mothers who are infected transmit the virus to their children. Among infants with HIV, in 79% of cases, one or both parents have been infected with the virus or have been members of a high-risk group. To date, AIDS has developed in about half the cases of HIV infection reported in children. Currently, the earliest that antibodies to HIV can be detected in infants is 15–18 months after birth, because infants may carry maternal antibodies rather than their own (passive immunity). After 6 months, an infant's own immune system begins to develop, and the level of maternal antibodies begins to decrease. At this time, the presence of HIV would trigger the infant's system to produce antibodies to the virus. A relatively new method is being used to detect HIV infection in infants who still carry antibodies from their mothers. A technique called polymerase chain reaction is used to detect viral DNA. When this method is used, the presence of HIV can be detected in infants as young as 3 months.

WHO IS AT HIGHEST RISK?

The following groups are at increased risk of becoming infected with HIV:

1. Homosexual and bisexual men who have multiple sexual partners, who have unprotected sex with a partner who is seropositive for HIV, and who engage in anal or oral intercourse (as an active or passive partner). Most reported cases of AIDS have been in homosexual men.

2. Heterosexual partners who have unprotected vaginal, anal, or oral intercourse with a partner who is seropositive for HIV. Thirty-five percent of cases of AIDS in women have been traced to sexual intercourse with an infected partner (Williams, 1992).

3. Children of women who are seropositive for HIV.

4. IDUs who share blood-contaminated needles.

Others who may still be at risk for HIV infection are those who receive blood transfusions or blood products. Currently, blood products used by hemophiliacs are heat-treated and tested for antibodies to HIV. Blood donated for transfusions is also tested for the presence of antibodies to HIV.

The screening procedures used by blood banks and plasma donor centers is a three-tiered exclusion process. It includes a detailed information sheet that lists multiple reasons for excluding a possible donor, an interview that reviews the material on the information sheet, and a bar-coded yes-no sheet. The bar-coded sheet was developed so that potential donors who think that disclosure would identify them as antibody-positive for HIV can still donate blood but have the blood discarded according to the information given by the bar code. The bar code cannot be visually read by blood bank personnel. The donor selects yes or no in privacy, and the remaining portions of the sheet are destroyed.

Finally, many states have adopted rigid regulations for notifying donors about the donors' HIV status. These regulations require a waiting period (6 months in California) before a person who is antibody positive for HIV can be notified. This is intended to discourage persons from donating blood or plasma in order to discover their antibody status. The waiting period further decreases the risk that donated blood will be infected with HIV.

Because of the window (time between infection and development of measurable antibodies), however, there is a slight risk that some donated blood will be infected, even after thorough screening and testing. Consequently, some patients prefer autologous transfusions, in which they receive their own blood. When they are planning to have a procedure in which a transfusion may be required, they donate blood beforehand and have it stored until needed. Fresh blood can be stored safely for 45 days, and frozen blood can be stored for 6 months. Those interested in receiving autologous transfusions should discuss the possibility with their physician. They should also check with their health insurance company to see if this method is covered under their policy. Many health insurance companies require payment for the transfusion even when it is the insured person's own blood.

HIV INFECTION AND HEALTH CARE WORKERS

As the number of persons infected with HIV increases, the prevalence of the infection in the health care environment will also increase. The risk of acquiring HIV infection as a health care worker has been the subject of conjecture, discussion, and research (Fischl et al., 1987). The risk from occupational exposure to persons infected with HIV has been evaluated at several medical centers and is the subject of ongoing study at the CDC. Studies of household contacts indicate that the risk to health care workers who have close personal contact with HIV-infected persons is extremely low (Becker, Cone, & Gerberding, 1989). A study of more than 4,000 health care workers exposed to body fluids potentially contaminated with HIV found that the risk of infection was less than 0.1% per year of exposure. This included more than 1,200 workers who had parenteral puncture wounds caused by contaminated needles or accidental splashes of blood on nonintact skin or mucous membranes,

As a matter of perspective, another blood-borne pathogen, HBV, is more dangerous than HIV to health care workers. However, it is not perceived as a threat by them. HBV is 100 times more infectious than HIV and causes more than 200 deaths each year among health care workers. Yet, HBV can be prevented by prophylaxis with hepatitis B vaccine before exposure to blood and blood products. Unfortunately, because many health care workers do not perceive themselves at risk, they do not obtain the vaccine (Lloyd, 1990).

In comparison, 65 cases of occupational transmission of HIV in health care workers have been reported. All the cases involved needle-stick injuries or splashes of contaminated body fluids on nonintact mucous membranes. The only body fluid implicated in transmission to health care workers has been blood or blood-contaminated fluid (Becker et al., 1989; Friedland & Klein, 1988; Gerberding, 1988). Health care workers at greatest risk are those who are regularly exposed to needles or other sharp objects while caring for patients.

The next chapter examines ways to prevent transmission of HIV in the health care setting and in our homes and community.

EXAM QUESTIONS

Chapter 2

Questions 8 - 12

8. HIV can be transmitted through which of the following?

    a. Urine, blood, vaginal secretions
    b. Urine, saliva, feces
    c. Blood, breast milk, saliva
    d. Blood, breast milk, semen

9. Which of the following is one reason injecting drug users are at risk for HIV infection?

    a. Bisexuality
    b. Heterosexuality
    c. Use of cocaine
    d. Sharing of contaminated needles and syringes

10. Which of the following behaviors most increase the risk of becoming infected with HIV?

    a. Using street drugs, having one sex partner
    b. Being a prostitute, using street drugs
    c. Sharing equipment for injecting drugs, becoming pregnant
    d. Sharing equipment for injecting drugs, having protected sex with multiple partners

11. When did screening of donated blood to prevent transmission of HIV infection begin in the United States?

    a. 1975
    b. 1985
    c. 1980
    d. 1990

12. Which of the following is a known way in which HIV is transmitted?

    a. Hugging a person who has AIDS
    b. Exposure to the sweat of someone infected with HIV
    c. Sexual intercourse with someone infected with HIV
    d. Donating blood

CHAPTER 3

PREVENTING TRANSMISSION OF HIV

CHAPTER OBJECTIVE

After studying this chapter, the reader will be able to describe practices that reduce the risk of becoming infected with HIV in the hospital setting and in the social environment.

LEARNING OBJECTIVES

After studying this chapter, the reader should be able to

1. Specify which patients should be presumed to have HIV infection.

2. Indicate situations in which gloves, masks, eye protection, and gowns or aprons should be worn.

3. Indicate when health care workers infected with HIV should refrain from direct care of patients.

4. Specify baseline laboratory tests that should be performed when a health care worker has an occupational exposure to HIV.

5. Indicate how long a hospital should monitor a health care worker who has had an occupational exposure to HIV.

6. Indicate which group in major cities has decreased its rate of HIV infection by changing its sexual practices.

7. Describe safe and unsafe sex practices.

8. Specify risk-reduction education that should be provided to patients to help prevent the transmission of HIV.

INTRODUCTION

In the early days of the AIDS epidemic, preventing transmission of HIV was a matter of great concern. As knowledge about HIV increased and epidemiologic studies delineated the routes of transmission, information was shared between the CDC, U.S. Public Health Service, and the National Institutes of Health (NIH). Because of this cooperative effort, the CDC, the federal Occupational Safety and Health Administration (OSHA), and other research and treatment groups have developed guidelines to prevent transmission of HIV through sexual activity, drug use, and occupational exposure (health care workers).

PREVENTING TRANSMISSION

Preventing the transmission of HIV is the responsibility of individuals, society, public health organizations, and the government. Nurses and educators in the health profession have a responsibility to ensure that every patient, friend, and relative knows and understands how HIV is transmitted and how transmission can be prevented. Sexually active persons and IDUs have a responsibility to themselves, their sexual partners, and their children to avoid activities that increase the risk of acquiring and transmitting HIV.

Education about HIV infection seems to be the key to eliminating myths about AIDS and to convincing some persons that AIDS is truly a disease, not a judgment. An important message that still has not been completely accepted is that HIV cannot be transmitted by casual contact.

In many areas, health agencies and the gay community have made an all-out effort to educate persons at risk about the dangers of multiple sexual partners and unsafe sex. To some degree, this has worked. The number of cases in homosexuals in certain cities, such as San Francisco, has decreased. However, HIV infection in teenagers, heterosexuals, and minority groups has become an increasing worry to public health officials. HIV infection and AIDS are often perceived as "gay white" diseases. A recent study showed that many heterosexuals continue to have multiple sexual partners and to have intercourse without condoms. In addition, because of religious and societal taboos, minority men may be reluctant to seek help. Many public health agencies are making a special effort to disseminate information about AIDS to Hispanics and blacks.

Sex and sexual activity have not been subjects of academic discussion in many nursing programs. However, the advent of HIV disease has made it imperative that nurses know and understand sexual terms and sexual activities. Patients' histories should include information on sexual activities and sexual partners so that appropriate education can be provided to every patient.

Sexual Transmission

Sexual transmission of HIV can be prevented or the risk of transmission decreased by adherence to the following sexual practices:

- Abstinence

- A mutually monogamous relationship

- Avoidance of anal or vaginal intercourse with anyone who is seropositive for HIV

- Use of latex condoms with nonoxynol-9 spermicide for insertive anal or vaginal intercourse

Homosexuals in major cities have shown that changes in sexual behaviors can affect the rate of infection with HIV, as well as the transmission of other sexually transmitted diseases such as gonorrhea and hepatitis B. However, among heterosexuals, widespread changes in sexual practices that increase the risk of transmission have not occurred. Therefore, nurses must educate everyone—heterosexuals, homosexuals, bisexuals, teenagers, children, and adults—about the risks of sex with multiple partners and the risks of unprotected intercourse. It is also important to counsel seropositive partners to use latex condoms and nonoxynol-9 during any intercourse activities to prevent the exchange of different types of HIV between partners.

Persons also need to know the risks related to oral sex and French kissing. Blood, semen, and vaginal secretions can contain high concentrations of HIV. Oral secretions do not contain large amounts of HIV. However, sores or cuts in the mouth or gum disease can result in bleeding or permit entry of the virus. For safer oral sex, dental dams, condoms, or nonmicrowaveable plastic wrap can be used during activities such as cunnilingus (oral stimulation of a female's genitals) or fellatio (oral stimulation or manipulation of the penis) (Wofsy, 1988).

Patients with HIV infection or AIDS will naturally want to know what they can do to make sex safer. Their family members will have questions, too. The Gay Men's Health Crisis (GMHC), an informational and support group for AIDS patients and their families and lovers, maintains that guidelines for safer sex are not just for patients who have AIDS. They are for everyone. This includes not only those who are infected with the virus (even if they are symptom-free) but also those who are not infected (National Gay Rights Advocates, 1986).

The GMHC suggests that one of the most important safeguards persons can follow is to know their sexual partner and their partner's sexual habits. Having multiple sexual partners increases the risk of becoming infected with HIV, as well as the risk of acquiring other sexually transmitted diseases.

Safe sex consists of activities in which no exchange of body fluids occurs. They include the following (AIDS Project/LA, 1986, 1988):

- Massage, hugging, cuddling, mutual masturbation

- Social kissing (kissing on cheeks or lips)

- Body-to-body rubbing (frottage), voyeurism, exhibitionism, fantasy

Unsafe sex is any physical contact that involves the exchange of body fluids or blood (Moon, 1986). Examples include the following:

- Receptive anal intercourse without a condom (receiving)

- Insertive anal intercourse without a condom (inserting)

- Insertion of the fist or any foreign object into the rectum ("fisting")

- Fellatio or orogenital contact without a barrier

- Oroanal stimulation ("rimming") without a barrier

- Vaginal intercourse without a condom

Despite warnings, some patients will continue to engage in unsafe sexual activities. The following are ways to reduce the risk of HIV transmission:

- Never swallow any body secretions, such as semen or vaginal secretions.

- Avoid direct contact with blood. The main way HIV is transmitted is through blood and semen.

- Avoid inserting objects into the rectum, vagina, or penis that might break the mucosa. HIV can enter the bloodstream through breaks in the mucosa.

- Avoid having sex with anonymous partners.

- Use latex condoms with nonoxynol-9 and a reservoir tip.

Suggestions for safer use of condoms (Kelly & St. Lawrence, 1987) include the following:

- Use a latex condom with a reservoir tip, to avoid direct contact with seminal fluid.

- Discard a condom after a single use.

- Use an uncontaminated, water-soluble lubricant. Do not use oil-based lubricants such as petroleum jelly or vegetable shortening.

- Use diaphragms and condoms in conjunction with water-soluble lubricants containing 5% nonoxynol-9. (Up to 50% of females are allergic to nonoxynol-9. It is recommended that females test the spermicide before using it during sexual activity. Those who have allergic reactions to it should not use it.)

Transmission via Needles or Drug Equipment

Transmission of HIV through sharing of needles is increasing. Drug users should not share needles or their equipment. According to Wofsy (1988), the message is, "Don't experiment with IV drugs; for users, get drug treatment; if using, don't share needles; clean your equipment (works); clean your skin; and avoid shooting galleries" (p. 311).

Sharing of drugs and needles is a social experience as well as a convenience. Therefore, methods to bring about changes in behavior must be culturally and ethically appropriate, and must involve the entire drug family and peer network. Needle exchange programs have been started in some cities to decrease the transmission of HIV through contaminated works. Opponents of these programs think that this practice promotes drug use and that other methods should be used. One effective method is to stress cleaning of the "works" (see Figure 8, p.31). Bleach is an effective, convenient, and cheap choice for doing this. A solution of 1 part bleach to 10 parts water kills viruses and inactivates HIV within 1 minute (Wofsy, 1988). The San Francisco AIDS Foundation and other organizations can provide more specific information on how to clean needles and other drug equipment.

Maternal Transmission

Maternal transmission of HIV to infants via the placenta, during birth, or via breast milk is also on the increase. Seventy-seven percent of children less than 13 years old who are infected with HIV have acquired the virus from their infected mother. In order to prevent this means of transmission, men and women at risk for HIV infection should be offered counseling and testing. Pregnant women who are infected should be provided information and counseling that will enable them to make decisions about childbearing issues (Wofsy, 1988).

INFECTION CONTROL IN THE HEALTH CARE SETTING

Infection control in the health care setting begins when a patient first seeks medical care. Hospitals now assume that any patient may be infected with HIV and are teaching health care workers to treat all patients as though the patients have a blood-borne infection. This includes the elderly, infants, and pregnant women. In addition, OSHA has adopted strict standards and rules for the prevention of occupational transmission of blood-borne pathogens, including HIV and HBV.

The CDC has recommended that all blood and body fluids be considered potentially infectious. When all

CHAPTER 3 —
PREVENTING TRANSMISSION OF HIV

31

Figure 8
CLEANING THE "WORKS"

THE BEST THING TO DO IS NOT SHOOT DRUGS! BUT IF YOU DO, YOU SHOULD ALWAYS USE CLEAN, NEW NEEDLES.

If you have to use someone else's works, first rinse the works a few times by pulling water up into syringe and squirting it out through the needle. Then do one of these three things to kill the AIDS virus.

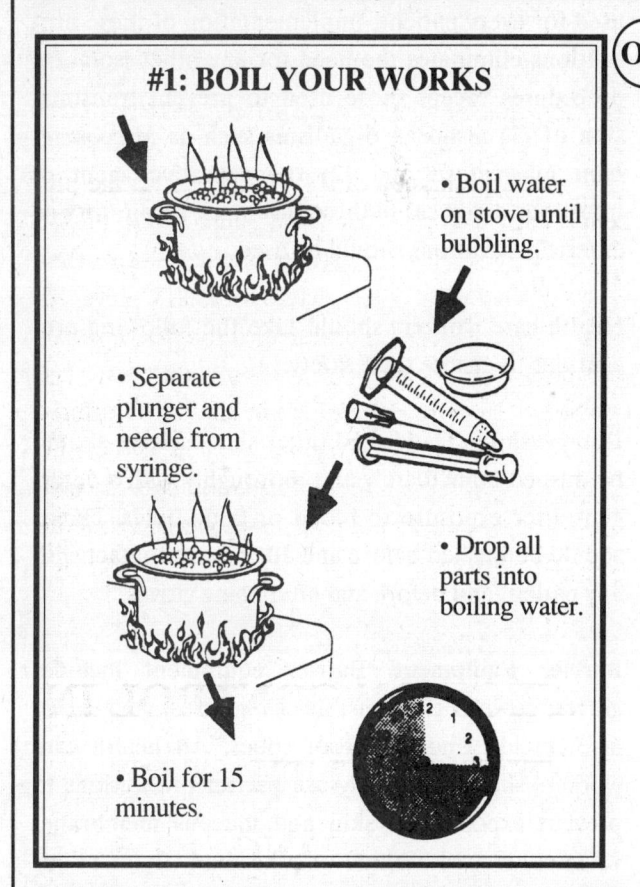

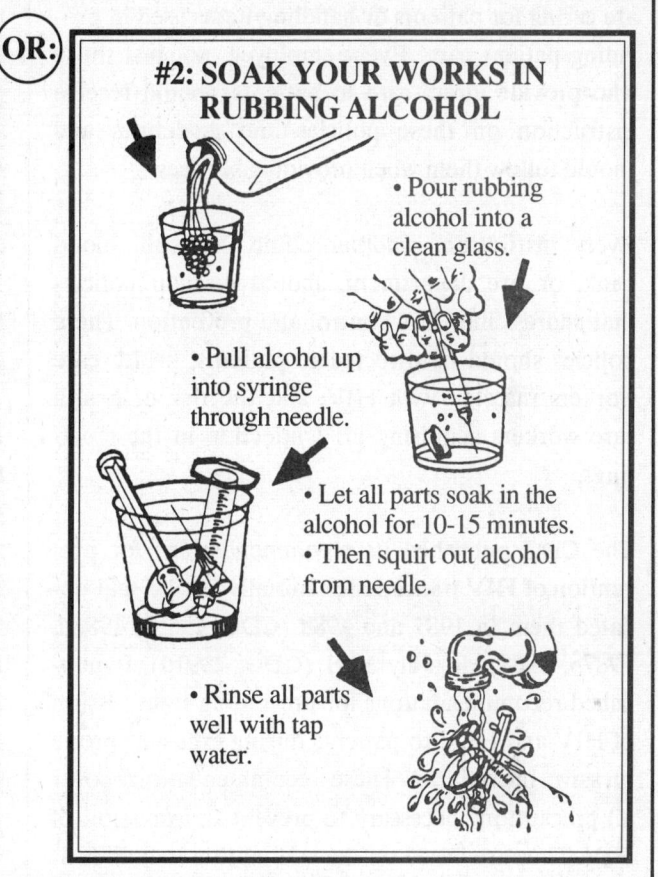

#1: BOIL YOUR WORKS

- Boil water on stove until bubbling.
- Separate plunger and needle from syringe.
- Drop all parts into boiling water.
- Boil for 15 minutes.

OR:

#2: SOAK YOUR WORKS IN RUBBING ALCOHOL

- Pour rubbing alcohol into a clean glass.
- Pull alcohol up into syringe through needle.
- Let all parts soak in the alcohol for 10-15 minutes.
- Then squirt out alcohol from needle.
- Rinse all parts well with tap water.

AIDS Foundation San Diego, 3777 4th Avenue, San Diego, California 92103 (619)543-0300

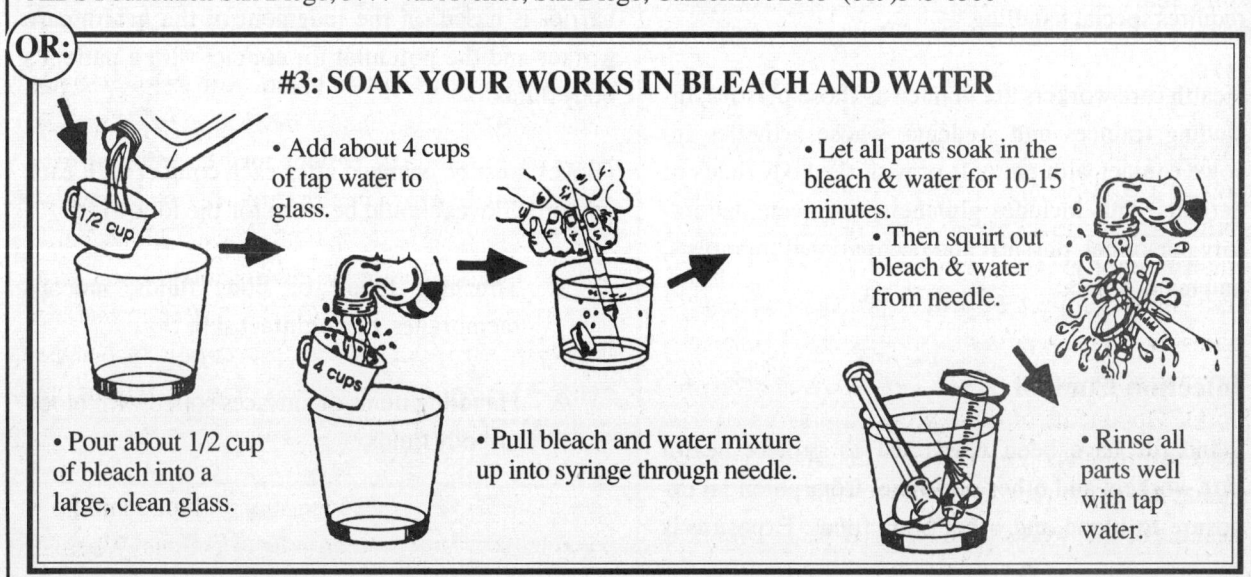

OR:

#3: SOAK YOUR WORKS IN BLEACH AND WATER

- Pour about 1/2 cup of bleach into a large, clean glass.
- Add about 4 cups of tap water to glass.
- Pull bleach and water mixture up into syringe through needle.
- Let all parts soak in the bleach & water for 10-15 minutes.
- Then squirt out bleach & water from needle.
- Rinse all parts well with tap water.

body fluids and secretions, including blood, are treated as potentially infectious, knowledge of special precautions is no longer required.

Each health care institution has established policies and guidelines for staff members to follow when they are caring for patients or handling items used in providing patient care. Every employee, not just those who provide direct care to patients, should receive instruction on these policies and guidelines and should follow them when providing services.

Every institution, whether clinic, hospital, blood bank, or fire department, should develop policies that address infection control and prevention. These policies should be directed to patients, health care workers infected with HIV, and the risk of health care workers acquiring HIV infection in these settings.

The CDC published its recommendations for prevention of HIV transmission initially in 1985 and updated them in 1987 and 1988 (CDC, 1985b, 1986d, 1987b, 1988). In July 1991 (CDC, 1991d), it published recommendations for preventing transmission of HIV and HBV to patients during exposure-prone invasive procedures. These recommendations cover all precautions necessary to prevent transmission of HIV. They are based on the assumption that all hospital waste that may be contaminated by body fluids requires special handling.

Health care workers are defined as those persons, including trainees and students, whose activities involve contact with patients or with the body fluids of patients. This includes plumbers, engineers, laboratory personnel, physical and occupational therapists, and many others.

Infection Control

Standards have been developed to protect health care workers and other personnel from potential exposure to blood and other body fluids. Exposure is best defined as contact with nonintact skin or mucous membranes.

The system of universal precautions is based on the assumption that everyone is potentially infectious. Therefore, handwashing and barrier precautions are used for every patient. Implementation of these precautions eliminates the need for any other isolation procedures except those used to prevent transmission of (1) airborne organisms such as *Mycobacterium tuberculosis* and (2) the causative agent of infectious diarrhea. In these instances, respiratory or enteric precautions should be used.

Health care workers should take the following precautions to ensure their safety:

Handwashing. Hands and other skin surfaces should be washed immediately and thoroughly with a detergent after exposure to blood or body fluids. Hands should be washed before and after every contact with any patient and before and after using gloves.

Barrier Equipment. Barrier equipment includes gloves; gowns or aprons; masks; glasses, goggles, or face shields; and leakproof shoes. All health care workers should routinely use barrier precautions to prevent exposure of skin and mucous membranes when contact with blood or other body fluids of any patient or person is likely. Use of the appropriate barrier is based on the judgment of the health care worker and the potential for contact with a patient's body fluids.

Gloves must be changed after each contact with each patient. Gloves should be worn for the following:

1. Touching blood or body fluids, mucous membranes, or nonintact skin

2. Handling items or surfaces soiled with blood or body fluids

CHAPTER 3 —
PREVENTING TRANSMISSION OF HIV

3. Performing venipuncture or other vascular access procedures

Gowns or aprons should be worn during procedures or activities in which contact with blood or body fluids may occur. This includes procedures that may generate droplets of blood or other body fluids. A different gown or apron should be worn for each patient contact, and gowns and aprons should be changed between each patient contact.

Masks should be worn whenever fluids or secretions may be produced from the respiratory system. This includes when a patient is coughing and when suctioning is required.

Glasses, goggles, or other protective eye wear such as face shields should be worn for procedures that may generate droplets of blood or other body fluids that could splash onto the face or into the eyes.

Disposable mouthpieces for emergency resuscitation procedures or other ventilation equipment should be readily available for use in all patient areas.

Disposal of Sharp Objects. Sharp objects, needles, and scalpels should be discarded into puncture-resistant containers. They should never be placed in paper or in trash. Uncapped needles should never be placed in beds, on trays, or in the trash. Recapped needles should never be put in the pocket of a uniform or coat or jacket. Recapping needles should be avoided. If a needle must be recapped, the one-hand recapping technique should be used (see Table 3).

Leakproof Containers. Specimens should be placed in leakproof containers such as closeable plastic bags. Any liquid waste should also be placed in leakproof containers.

Waste Disposal. HIV-infected wastes as well as other pathologic waste should be handled according to policies and procedures consistent with local and state health regulations. All biological wastes from the pathology department should be autoclaved or incinerated.

Table 3
ONE-HAND RECAPPING TECHNIQUE

Use the following procedure when needles or sharp objects cannot be disposed of or must be carried to another room or when the needle must be removed from a syringe or other piece of equipment.

1. Remove the cap of the needle or the cover of the sharp object and place it on a firm surface on its side.

2. When planned procedure or activity is completed, use one hand to slip the needle or sharp object completely into the cap or cover on the firm surface.

3. Do not use the free hand to hold the cap or cover.

4. Secure the cap or cover on the needle or sharp object by grasping the base of the cap or cover.

5. Place the capped needle or covered sharp object in a puncture-proof container.

Laundry. Soiled linen should be handled as little as possible. It should be placed in a container in the room where it has been used and then transported.

The CDC has also outlined appropriate precautions to be used by dentists, pathologists, and morticians and in dialysis centers and laboratories. Specifics for these precautions can be found in the *MMWR* supplement for August 21, 1987 (CDC, 1987c).

Finally, health care workers with exudative lesions or open cuts should refrain from all direct patient care and from handling equipment used in patient care. Health care workers with respiratory infections should also refrain from direct patient care, and all health care workers should be immunized against influenza every fall. Health care workers who are seropositive for HIV should be aware of the potential for transmission of HIV to their patients and other workers.

HEALTH CARE WORKERS AND HIV

To maintain the integrity of medical care for those infected with HIV and to protect the rights of health care workers, institutions must consider the legal and ethical questions raised by fear of occupational exposure. The ongoing debate and controversy about occupational transmission of HIV has two aspects: (1) transmission from an infected patient to an uninfected health care worker and (2) transmission from an infected health care worker to an uninfected patient (Brennan, 1991).

Health care workers who work with needles and sharp objects and who provide direct care are the most at risk for occupational exposure to HIV. The estimated risk of infection with HIV after a percutaneous injury by a needle or sharp object is 0.3% for all health care workers. The risk of potential infection after exposure via the skin or mucous membranes is highest in areas where large numbers of HIV-infected persons live. The risk also increases when invasive procedures are performed and is higher in hospital units that have a high proportion of HIV-infected patients.

In response to increasing concerns of health care workers, the American Nurses' Association (ANA), health care institutions, and the government have increased efforts to inform health care workers about HIV and other blood-borne pathogens, including transmission and prevention of transmission.

Health care workers need orientation and continuing education and training on how to prevent exposure to blood and body fluids. This must cover epidemiology, modes of transmission, and ways to prevent transmission of HIV and other blood-borne pathogens. Use of universal precautions for all patients should be stressed. Emphasis should be placed on proper disposal of needles, scalpels, and sharp objects.

All health care facilities must have established policies on procedures to be followed when a health care worker has an occupational exposure to HIV. A policy on the distribution of zidovudine (azidothymidine [AZT], Retrovir) to employees who have been exposed to blood and body fluids should also be established.

Employees who have been or may have been exposed to HIV should be counseled on the risks involved and encouraged to have baseline laboratory tests. These include tests for antibodies to HIV, screening for hepatitis B, VDRL tests, and liver function tests. Testing of the source patient whose HIV status is unknown is now recommended if the employer plans on providing zidovudine to workers who have had an occupational exposure. Additional tests for antibodies to HIV and hepatitis B screening should be done 6–12 weeks after the exposure. In some situations, tests for antibodies to HIV may also be repeated at 6 months and 12 months after the exposure.

CDC recommendations (1990b) for the use of zidovudine in health care workers who have had an occupational exposure to HIV are as follows: The worker should be given four capsules of zidovudine (100 mg each) immediately (preferably within 30 minutes) and then two capsules every 4 hour five times a day for 1 month. If the HIV status of the patient is unknown, the health care worker should take zidovudine until the status of the patient is known. If

CHAPTER 3 —
PREVENTING TRANSMISSION OF HIV

the patient is seronegative for HIV antibodies, the drug should be stopped. If the patient is seropositive, treatment with zidovudine should be continued for 1 month.

Counseling of the injured employee should cover risks of HIV infection, how to prevent potential exposure of sexual partners, risks and benefits of HIV antibody testing, instructions to report any acute febrile illness that occurs within 12 weeks of the exposure, and follow-up procedures. Employees should be monitored (if they desire) for 3–6 months after the exposure and provided with appropriate emotional and psychologic support.

The same precautions and considerations should be taken when a patient is exposed to the blood or body fluids of a health care worker. The patient should be informed of the incident and counseled the same way employees are counseled. Appropriate testing should be offered, as well as zidovudine when it is appropriate.

In addition to its requirements for education, provision of equipment, and health care should an injury occur, OSHA has issued a blood-borne pathogen standard that took effect in March 1992 (Howe, 1992a; "New OSHA Guidelines," 1992). This standard mandates hospitals, clinics, and other employers, including doctors' and dentists' offices, to protect employees against accidental exposure to HIV and HBV or face fines of up to $70,000.

The standard provides wide-ranging workplace protections for health care workers who may have occupational exposure to HIV and HBV. Employers must establish a written exposure-control plan and provide free hepatitis vaccinations, puncture-resistant containers for needles and sharp objects, personal protective equipment, training, and medical surveillance. Additional information about this new OSHA standard can be obtained from local OSHA offices or by calling the federal OSHA office: (202) 523-8151.

Adding to the controversy and dilemmas associated with the care of HIV-infected patients are continuing efforts by some for mandatory HIV testing of all hospital patients. Few authorities have supported this type of testing because of the cost involved, lack of guidelines for the frequency of testing, and the recognition that knowing a patient's HIV status does not protect the health care worker.

Just what is the risk that an employee will become infected with HIV in the health care setting? The CDC recently reported that health care workers in the United States were not becoming infected with the virus at abnormally high rates ("CDC Reports Few," 1992). As of June 1990, health care workers accounted for less than 5% of the 137,385 adults and adolescents known to have AIDS. Of these workers, 94% had a history of other risk factors such as unsafe sexual activities, use of injectable drugs, or blood transfusions.

The identification of five persons who may have become infected while receiving care from an infected dentist created a public outcry for mandatory HIV testing and the demand that patients be informed about the HIV status of health care workers. In response to this outcry, Senator Jessie Helms (R-North Carolina) sponsored an amendment that was passed by the United States Senate. It would have required that patients be informed about a health care worker's HIV status before any exposure-prone invasive procedures are done. The amendment further proposed a fine of $10,000 and 10 years imprisonment for noncompliance ("Helms Amendment," 1991). The CDC responded to the outcry by proposing a plan to list procedures that HIV-infected health care workers should not perform ("Public Education Defuses," 1991). These measures led to further controversy and to outcries from nurses, physicians, and dentists across the nation. After much discussion and debate, Senator Helm's amendment and the CDC proposal were dropped.

However, the controversy has not ended. Requests for mandatory testing of patients and health care workers continue. It should be recognized that mandatory HIV testing would do nothing to prevent transmission from patient to worker, worker to patient, or patient to patient. Use of universal precautions is the best way to prevent transmission of HIV in the health care setting.

Mandatory HIV testing is not a form of infection control. The tests detect only the presence of antibodies, which may take months to develop. During those months, the infected person can transmit the virus, yet tests for antibodies to HIV are negative. Finally, mandatory testing is extremely expensive. The estimated annual expense is $1 million. This money would be better spent on education on how to prevent HIV infection and on early intervention when infection occurs ("Public Education Defuses," 1991).

Finally, nurses as health care workers should take every advantage to be informed about HIV infection, transmission of the virus, prevention of transmission, and legal and political issues. The ANA is one source of information. Over the years, it has adopted more than 20 policies and position statements related to HIV infection and AIDS. These include position statements on HIV testing, programs that should be followed if occupational exposure to HIV or HBV occurs, and personnel policies and HIV in the workplace ("ANA Statements Focus," 1991). For additional information on health care workers and HIV, see CDC, 1987c; Gerberding, 1988; and Jackson et al., 1987.

The next chapter discusses HIV disease in women.

EXAM QUESTIONS

Chapter 3

Questions 13 - 21

13. Among persons seeking health care, which of the following should be presumed to have HIV infection?

    a. Surgical patients only
    b. Homosexual men only
    c. Injecting drug users only
    (d.) All patients

14. In addition to gowns and gloves, what kind of protection should be used during procedures that generate droplets or splashes of body fluids?

    a. Eyeglasses and protective footwear
    b. Mask and protective footwear
    c. Mask and double gloves
    (d.) Mask and protective face shield

15. Changes in behavior have led to a decrease in the rate of HIV infection in which of the following groups?

    (a.) Injecting drug users
    b. Pregnant women
    c. Heterosexuals
    d. Homosexual men

16. How long should health care workers who have had a needle-stick injury or splash exposure to HIV be monitored?

    a. 1–2 weeks
    b. 3–6 weeks
    c. 1–2 months
    (d.) 3–6 months

17. Health care workers should refrain from providing direct patient care when they have which of the following?

    a. Diarrhea
    b. Antibodies to HIV
    c. Antibodies to hepatitis B virus
    (d.) Open cuts or exudative sores

18. Which of the following is considered a safe sex practice?

    a. Anal intercourse
    (b.) Mutual masturbation
    c. Oral sex
    d. Vaginal intercourse

19. Baseline laboratory tests that should be done when a health care worker has had a needle-stick injury or splash exposure to HIV include tests for antibodies to HIV and:

    (a.) Screening for hepatitis B virus
    b. Skin tests for *Mycobacterium tuberculosis*
    c. Pulmonary function tests
    d. B-cell count

20. Which of the following is considered an unsafe sex practice?

    a. Frottage
    b. Mutual masturbation
    (c.) Unprotected vaginal or anal intercourse
    d. Kissing

21. What type of barrier protection should be worn when handling infectious material and body fluids and splashing is not anticipated?

    a. Mask and gown
    b. Gown
    c. Gloves
    d. Eyeglasses or mask

CHAPTER 4

HIV DISEASE IN WOMEN

CHAPTER OBJECTIVE

After studying this chapter, the reader will be able to discuss epidemiologic findings, assessment procedures, and common problems associated with HIV disease in women.

LEARNING OBJECTIVES

After studying this chapter, the reader should be able to

1. Specify the prevalence of AIDS in women in the United States.

2. Indicate the most frequent mode of transmission of HIV in women.

3. Specify the factors that probably account for the number of AIDS cases detected in women.

4. Describe the most common problems encountered by women who have AIDS.

5. Specify the information nurses should request during an interview with a woman who may have HIV disease.

6. Specify the educational information that should be given to women who are infected with HIV or are at risk for infection with HIV.

INTRODUCTION

HIV disease has affected women since 1981, not only because they are sexual partners and IDUs but also because they are mothers and the major group of people who provide health care. As of February 1992, AIDS had been diagnosed in 22,056 women. The rate of increase in the number of cases was 29%, as compared with 18% in men. Women now account for more than 11% of all AIDS cases reported in the United States (Minkoff & DeHovitz, 1991; Williams, 1992). Many more women are at risk of acquiring HIV, and many of childbearing age are at risk of transmitting the virus to their offspring (CDC, 1990a).

Figure 9
WOMEN AND AIDS

Black and Hispanic women in their childbearing years account for a disproportionate number of the AIDS cases among women. The following charts illustrate the differences by comparing the estimated population distribution of women ages 15 to 44 with the distribution of AIDS cases among women of those ages.

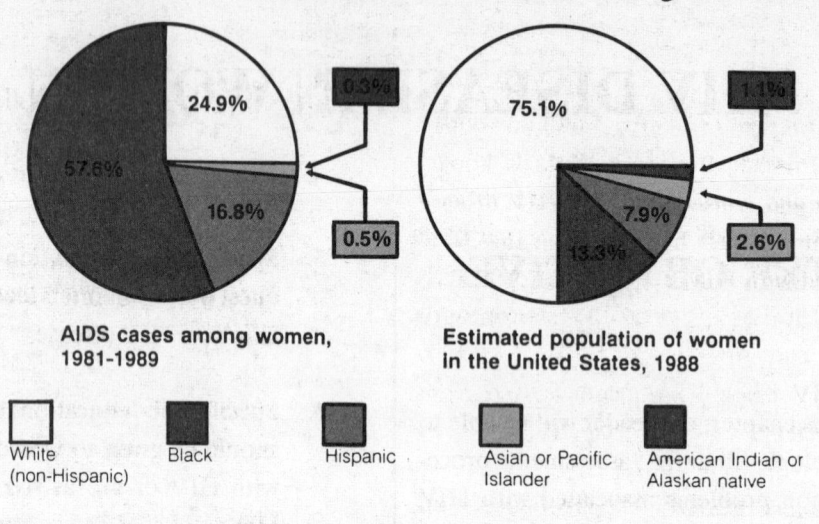

AIDS cases among women, 1981-1989
- White (non-Hispanic): 24.9%
- Black: 57.6%
- Hispanic: 16.8%
- Asian or Pacific Islander: 0.3%
- American Indian or Alaskan native: 0.5%

Estimated population of women in the United States, 1988
- White (non-Hispanic): 75.1%
- Black: 13.3%
- Hispanic: 7.9%
- Asian or Pacific Islander: 1.1%
- American Indian or Alaskan native: 2.6%

EPIDEMIOLOGY

In 1989, more than 35,000 persons who fit the case definition for AIDS were identified in the United States. Of these, almost 4,000 were women. The only transmission category in which women outnumber men is heterosexual contact. Women most frequently acquire HIV through drug use, via contaminated needles or drug equipment. Approximately 90% of all women with AIDS are 20–50 years old, and 71% have been IDUs or sexual partners of IDUs (Minkoff & DeHovitz, 1991; Williams, 1992). Black women account for 58% of the cases, and Hispanic women account for 17% (see Figure 9). One reason for this disproportionate distribution may be the high prevalence of IDUs in New York and Florida (Poole, 1988). In addition, more women than men have no identifiable risk, perhaps because a woman may not be aware of her exposure to a person in a high-risk group (Guinan & Hardy, 1987). Finally, the number of cases in children is on the increase because the majority of women with AIDS are in their childbearing years ("Being Alive," 1991).

Leibowitz (1989) attributes the increase in the number of women with AIDS to the following factors:

1. More men than women are infected with HIV. Therefore, women have an increased chance of contact with an infected sexual partner.

2. Male-to-female transmission is more efficient than female-to-male transmission.

3. Women appear to be less aware of the potential that their heterosexual or bisexual partner is infected or may be at risk of infection.

CHAPTER 4 —
HIV DISEASE IN WOMEN

4. Potentially, a woman is more likely than a man to have a traumatic sexual experience during heterosexual intercourse.

ASSESSMENT

Although worldwide an estimated 3 million women will die of AIDS during the 1990s, little is known about the course and consequences of HIV disease in women. Williams (1992) has suggested that 65% of women infected with HIV will die before AIDS is diagnosed. Little also is known about the appropriate standards of care for women. Most of what is known about HIV disease has been derived from men who are infected.

Gender may influence the social and biological consequences of HIV disease. Access to care may be different for women and men. Women are more likely to rely on clinic care or drug rehabilitation services. Full-service or primary health care for women is rare (Minkoff & DeHovitz, 1991; Williams, 1991). The pharmacologic effects of drugs may also vary with gender.

Because of these suspected and documented differences between men and women with HIV disease, nurses must be careful not to base decisions about care solely on information gathered about men with the disease. All women should be assessed for their risk for HIV infection, especially women who are treated for sexually transmitted diseases and women who are seen in pregnancy prevention programs, for prenatal examinations, or for routine gynecologic examinations.

A thorough history that addresses HIV risk factors is essential. Information about past and present health care problems and a thorough social history are also important. A thorough menstrual history is helpful as well, because women with immunosuppression can have abnormalities in their menstrual cycle.

Nurses must become comfortable obtaining sexual histories, and they must learn to ask questions in a nonthreatening, nonjudgmental, information-seeking manner. Maintaining confidentiality is also important.

Questions should include the following:

- Are you sexually active? If so, is your current partner your only partner?

- Have you had other partners in the past? When?

- Have you ever had gonorrhea, syphilis, or any other sexually transmitted disease?

- Have you ever been tested for or concerned about HIV infection? If so, when and what were the results?

- Have you ever had sex with someone at risk for HIV infection?

- Have you ever injected drugs into your body or shared needles with anyone?

- Have you ever had a blood transfusion? If so, when?

- Have you ever been artificially inseminated in order to become pregnant?

- Do you have any reason to suspect that you have been exposed to HIV?

After a complete history has been obtained, attention should be directed to physical findings that might indicate a woman is infected with HIV. Common indications include thrush, chronic vaginal candidiasis, or other infections; needle marks on arms, legs, neck, and breasts; nutritional status; skin problems; and respiratory problems (Poole, 1988).

Some of the signs and symptoms characteristic of HIV infection are similar in women and men. However, important differences exist. The most frequent initial sign in women is vaginal candidiasis or yeast infections that recur and require aggressive treatment. Kaposi's sarcoma is rarely seen in women, and, as in men, the prevalence of PCP has decreased. The CDC has recently recognized the differences faced by women with HIV disease. The definition of AIDS (CDC, 1992c) has been changed to include cervical cancer, which is being detected more often in women infected with HIV.

HIV DISEASE IN WOMEN

To date, few well-controlled studies on AIDS-defining illnesses in HIV-positive women have been done. Only recently have the course and consequences of HIV disease among women been better understood. Current information suggests that women who are seropositive for HIV are at greater risk for *Candida* esophagitis, infections caused by herpes simplex virus (HSV), and malignant epithelial tumors. Mucosal *Candida* infections, such as vaginitis, thrush, and esophagitis, are often the first indication that a woman is infected with HIV. Women with HIV disease also have an increased prevalence of human papillomavirus (HPV) infections, cervical neoplasia, and abnormal findings on Pap tests.

Women who are seropositive for HIV also have more gynecologic infections than women who are seronegative. Those who have pelvic inflammatory disease are likely to have more abscesses and require more surgical interventions. Vaginal candidiasis is often recurrent, and oral therapy with ketoconazole may be necessary when standard topical antifungal medications fail. The typical regimen is 400 mg of ketoconazole each day for 14 days and then a 5-day course each month for 6 months (Minkoff & DeHovitz, 1991).

Seropositive women may have unique manifestations of genital ulcers, which may not respond to acyclovir or syphilis therapy. Those who have HSV infections may also have more frequent shedding of HSV during the latter part of pregnancy. The herpetic ulcers may take longer to resolve, and long-term use of acyclovir may be needed. Finally, syphilis may be more aggressive in seropositive women, and neurosyphilis may occur (Williams, 1992).

Infection with HPV, a major cause of cervical cancer, is more often associated with cervical dysplasia in women who are seropositive for HIV. Infection with HPV can lead to genital warts (condyloma acuminata, vaginal and cervical lesions called flat warts), dysplasia, cervical and anal neoplasia, and invasive cancers. The reason for the increase in cervical dysplasia and neoplasia is not clear. Some think the immunosuppression associated with HIV infection makes the HPV infection worse. Evidence indicates that women with HIV infection who have low CD4 counts may be at increased risk for the development of cervical abnormalities. Therefore, it is recommended that women who are HIV positive have Pap smears every 6 months and culdoscopy if the Pap smear shows any abnormalities (Williams, 1992; Wilson & Lein, 1992).

To date, no evidence suggests that nongynecologic opportunistic infections other than *Candida* esophagitis are more prevalent in women who are seropositive for HIV. As the CD4 count drops below 300 cells/mm^3, the prevalence of *Candida* esophagitis increases. Treatment for this infection is the same for women and men.

Currently, treatment of HIV-related opportunistic infections and the response to and the effects of zidovudine treatment of HIV infections are the same for women and men. However, use of zidovudine in female IDUs has not been studied (Minkoff & DeHovitz, 1991).

PREGNANCY

Eighty-five percent of all HIV infections and cases of AIDS in women occur in women of childbearing age (Porcher, 1992). Determining a pregnant woman's risk of being infected or becoming infected with HIV is important. Often, the first indication that a women is HIV positive is the diagnosis of HIV infection in her newborn infant.

Women who are considering becoming pregnant or who are already pregnant should be educated about the risk of HIV infection to themselves and their unborn children. All women should be offered the opportunity before and after they become pregnant to have tests for HIV antibodies. To assist health care professionals in counseling women, the CDC (1985b) has published recommendations on how to prevent maternal transmission of HIV.

In January 1991, an Institute of Medicine panel recommended that HIV testing be offered to all pregnant women in areas where the prevalence of HIV infection is high. HIV screening should be voluntary, and written consent should be obtained from the patient before the tests are done (Williams, 1991). Health care providers should be aware that the results of these tests may be false-positive or indeterminate in pregnant women. The tests should be repeated if the results are indeterminate.

An HIV-infected mother has a 25–35% chance of transmitting the virus to her fetus or newborn infant. The virus can be transmitted in utero or during birth. (See chapter 5 for further discussion of HIV infections in infants.)

Knowledge of the HIV status of the mother will help both the mother and the baby, as some evidence indicates that zidovudine may protect the baby in utero. However, zidovudine is not licensed for use in pregnant women. The drug readily crosses the placenta, and data on its effects on the fetus are incomplete (Porcher, 1992).

Also, HIV infection may be affected by pregnancy. Some evidence suggests that women who are seropositive for HIV have rapid progression of their disease and increased mortality when they are pregnant. Research has shown that the high level of sex hormones, particularly progesterone, that exists during pregnancy induces a state of immunosuppression. Pregnancy also has been associated with alterations in immune function and changes in the ratio of CD4 to CD8 cells in women without HIV infection. Thus, further immunosuppression might occur in an HIV-infected woman during pregnancy, especially if the woman has symptomatic HIV infection or AIDS. Increased immunosuppression may accelerate the disease (Wilson & Lein, 1992).

COUNSELING AND GUIDELINES FOR SAFE SEX

Nurses should be prepared to counsel women on activities that prevent transmission of HIV or decrease the risk of becoming infected with the virus. The following recommendations can be given:

- Know your sex partner(s). Ask questions about past sexual activities and drug use.

- Unless you know your partner is not infected, do not permit your partner's blood (including menstrual blood), semen, vaginal secretions, urine, or feces to enter your vagina, anus, or mouth.

- Make male partners wear condoms during vaginal, anal, and oral sex.

- Use nonoxynol-9 contraceptive foams, jellies, or creams during vaginal and anal intercourse.

The nurse's role in preventing transmission of HIV cannot be minimized. Appropriate education to gay men in San Francisco drastically reduced the prevalence of HIV infection and the eventual development of AIDS. However, no similar education has been provided to women at risk for HIV disease. One reason is that most of the women who are infected with HIV are black or Hispanic. Efforts to avoid stigmatizing these two groups may have resulted in them denying their risk. Education done to illustrate the risk of heterosexual transmission featured white teenagers, white women, and white couples (Wofsy, 1987). In addition, early reports portrayed AIDS as a gay disease, not a disease of heterosexuals. Most recently, some reports have suggested that the risk of heterosexual transmission indicated by the CDC is greater than the actual risk. All these factors have led women, especially black and Hispanic women, to believe that they are not at risk for HIV infection.

ISSUES AFFECTING WOMEN WHO HAVE HIV DISEASE

Many issues must be confronted by women who are infected with HIV or are the significant other of someone infected with HIV. Women who are infected or who provide care to someone who is infected are frequently isolated. This isolation may be self-imposed because of the fear of discrimination, loss of social contact, or loss of acceptable physical attractiveness. As care providers, they may be embarrassed by the stigma of the disease or be unable to leave the home because of the infected person's requirements for care (Wofsy, 1987).

For women infected with HIV, sexual expression may be limited. Revealing that they are seropositive for HIV may destroy any existing relationships or ones just beginning. Many women's perceptions of themselves revolve around their roles of sexual partner and child bearer. Loss of these roles frequently leads to loss of self-esteem and problems with body image. These losses may be even more pronounced in IDUs, for whom drug use may be associated with problems with self-image.

Women, in general, have been the primary homemakers and parents for their families. HIV-infected women may have trouble fulfilling their responsibilities as parents, breadwinners, chief cooks, housekeepers, and so forth. They may experience guilt over having a child who has HIV disease, or they may have difficulty making plans for their surviving children. Feelings of anger, anxiety, hopelessness, and depression may be present because of fears and uncertainty. These feelings need to be addressed, and counseling and support provided.

Finally, finding physicians, obstetricians, gynecologists, sex counselors, abortion counselors, and health counselors who are familiar with issues related to HIV infection in women may be difficult. Many of these professionals themselves have not yet recognized that women are at risk, and so neglect to routinely include questions about HIV or tests for the virus (Wofsy, 1987).

HIV disease is a major public health epidemic. If predictions are accurate about the rate of HIV infection and the eventual development of AIDS in those infected, then the epidemic will only continue to

CHAPTER 4 —
HIV DISEASE IN WOMEN

grow. As it does, so will the number of women and children who are infected. Because of this growth, nurses and other members of society must take a more active part in preventing the transmission of HIV. They can be educators and help reduce behaviors that increase the risk of becoming infected.

The next chapter discusses the issues and problems of HIV infection and AIDS in infants, children, and adolescents.

EXAM QUESTIONS

Chapter 4

Questions 22 - 27

22. Women with AIDS have the most difficulty with which of the following problems?

    a. Isolation
    b. HIV-positive male partners
    c. Baby sitters
    d. Employment

23. What type of information is elicited by questions about sexual, menstrual, and pregnancy history; HIV risk factors; and sexually transmitted diseases?

    a. Woman-specific
    b. Sexually explicit
    c. Nonthreatening
    d. Routine medical

24. When discussing HIV infection, nurses should be prepared to educate and counsel women about all of the following except:

    a. Having sex with HIV-negative partners only
    b. Use of birth control methods
    c. Progression of HIV disease
    d. Preventing acquisition and transmission of HIV

25. Which of the following is frequently the first indicator of the presence of HIV infection in women?

    a. Pneumocystis pneumonia
    b. Mucosal candidiasis
    c. Recurrent pneumonia
    d. Pregnancy

26. Which of the following is one reason given for the increasing number of women with AIDS?

    a. Contact with a male partner
    b. Greater efficiency of male-to-female transmission
    c. Potential for having a transfusion after giving birth
    d. Drug use and prostitution

27. What is the most frequent mode of HIV transmission in women?

    a. Having sexual intercourse with an HIV-positive partner
    b. Sharing contaminated needles and syringes
    c. Giving birth to an HIV-positive infant
    d. Providing health care for someone who is HIV positive

CHAPTER 5

HIV DISEASE IN INFANTS, CHILDREN, AND ADOLESCENTS

CHAPTER OBJECTIVE

After studying this chapter, the reader will be able to describe differences and similarities between HIV infection and AIDS in adults and in infants and children.

LEARNING OBJECTIVES

After studying this chapter, the reader should be able to

1. Specify the rate of in utero transmission of HIV.

2. Indicate the most important risk factors for transmission of HIV among teenagers.

3. Specify two socioeconomic reasons why AIDS and HIV infection have become so prevalent in the United States.

4. Specify the age at which infants begin to produce their own immunoglobulins.

5. Indicate the age at which the results of HIV serologic tests are reliable in infants and children.

6. Recognize the indications for a computed tomography (CT) scan of the head of an infant or child.

7. Describe the more common clinical manifestations of HIV infection in infants and children.

8. Specify three criteria for diagnosis of HIV infection in infants or children.

9. Specify the most common clinical sign of HIV infection in infants infected in utero or during birth.

10. Indicate the immunizations an HIV-infected child should receive.

11. List the three goals for medical management of HIV infection and AIDS in infants and children.

12. Specify the most common nutritional problems of children who are infected with HIV.

13. Describe the differences between HIV infection in adults and HIV infection in infants and children.

14. Name the drug(s) used to modify the immune system of infants or children who have HIV infection.

15. Indicate the most common psychosocial issues associated with HIV infection in infants and children.

16. Specify the most important issues associated with the transmission of HIV in infants and children.

17. Indicate the reasons adolescents are at increased risk for HIV infection.

18. Suggest an approach for obtaining information about risk factors from an adolescent.

19. Describe the major psychosocial issues of adolescents who are infected with HIV.

INTRODUCTION

Like all other major infectious diseases, HIV disease has not been restricted to adults. Infants, children, and adolescents are also affected. HIV disease in these younger groups is both similar to and different from HIV disease in adults. This chapter focuses on the epidemiology, immunology, clinical care, social ramifications, and emotional consequences of HIV infection and AIDS in infants, children, and adolescents.

INFANTS AND CHILDREN

Epidemiology

Unknown before 1981, AIDS is rapidly becoming the leading cause of death among children (Novello, Wise, Willoughby, & Pizzo, 1989). By the end of 1985, children less than 13 years old accounted for 183 cases of AIDS diagnosed in the United States (Thurber & Berry, 1990). This number has increased steadily: 2,055 cases had been diagnosed by January 1990 ("Statistics," 1990), 3,426 by the end of November 1991 (CDC, 1992a), and 4,051 by September 1992 (CDC, 1992c).

These figures, however, severely underestimate the scope of the problem. Exposure during birth accounts for approximately 80% of the cases of HIV disease in infants and children. In 1988–1989, this route of transmission accounted for the second largest increase in the number of cases diagnosed (CDC, 1990b). Many women are unaware they are infected with HIV until HIV disease is diagnosed in their infant. Approximately 100,000 women of childbearing age in the United States are seropositive for HIV. The rate of maternal transmission of the virus is 20–35%. Potentially, any pregnant woman who is infected with HIV could transmit the virus to her infant in utero or during birth (Bernstein et al., 1989; Thurber & Berry, 1990). On the basis of these statistics, more than 20,000 children in the United States may currently be infected with HIV.

Most of the infants and children who have HIV disease are black or Hispanic. Although only 15% of children in the United States are black and only 10% are Hispanic, black children account for 53% of AIDS cases in this age group, and Hispanic children account for 22% (Novello et al., 1989). These figures show that the ramifications for future generations of blacks and Hispanics will be enormous and tragic (Lauerman, 1989).

CHAPTER 5 —
HIV DISEASE IN INFANTS, CHILDREN, AND ADOLESCENTS

Table 4
CRITERIA FOR DIAGNOSIS OF HIV INFECTION IN CHILDREN

I. Children under 15 months old with perinatal HIV antibody must have one of the following:

- HIV present in blood or tissue
- Symptoms meeting CDC case definition of AIDS
- Evidence of cellular or humoral immunodeficiency
- Symptomatic infection (failure to thrive, lymphadenopathy, progressive neurologic disease, lymphoid interstitial pneumonitis, secondary infections of AIDS definition)
- Symptoms meeting CDC definition of AIDS

II. Older perinatally infected children or those who acquired infection by transfusions or sexual abuse must have one of the following:

- HIV in blood or tissues
- HIV antibody
- Symptoms meeting CDC definition of AIDS

Source: Centers for Disease Control, 1987a.

According to Bernstein et al. (1989), two reasons explain why HIV disease is becoming more prevalent in the United States: poverty and drug abuse. They state that until realistic options for dealing with these two major issues become available, HIV disease among women and children will continue.

Immunology, Serology, and Testing

The effect of HIV infection on the immune system of an infant or child is different from its effect on the immune system of an adult. Newborns and infants have an immature immune system that becomes competent over time. Although the total level of antibodies or immunoglobulins may be high (hypergammaglobulinemia) in infants and children infected with HIV, the immune system in these two age groups is not very effective at producing antibodies against a specific infecting organism.

Serologic testing for HIV in infants is unreliable for several months after birth because maternal antibodies cross the placenta. If a pregnant woman is seropositive for HIV, her antibodies against the virus will cross the placenta and be present in her infant when the child is born. For approximately 18 months after birth, antibodies produced by the infant cannot be distinguished from antibodies the infant received in utero from the mother.

Infants begin to produce their own immunoglobulin about 4–6 months after birth. Lack of antibody at 6 months could indicate that the infant's immune system is impaired. Some infants who have been infected in utero are never able to make antibody because their immune system is so incompetent.

The most reliable diagnosis of HIV infection in infants is based on tests that indicate the virus is present in the blood or tissues. These include culture of the virus or detection of viral DNA by using the polymerase chain reaction. Immunodeficiency is indicated by an increase in the level of immunoglobulins, a decrease in the CD4 count, and a decrease in the ratio of CD4 to CD8 T cells or absolute lymphopenia (Arpadi & Caspe, 1990). Tests to detect the virus (rather than antibodies to the virus) are expensive, however. Therefore, until proved otherwise, all infants whose mothers have antibodies to HIV are assumed to be seropositive for the virus. Care of the infant is then directed toward prevention of complications (Arpadi & Caspe, 1990; Bernstein et al., 1989; Thurber & Berry, 1990).

Table 4 (p.49) gives the CDC criteria for diagnosis of HIV infection in infants and children.

DEFINITION OF HIV DISEASE IN CHILDREN

Recognition of AIDS in children led to the development of the case definition of the syndrome in infants and children for surveillance purposes. Early definitions were too restrictive to provide a valid indication of the extent of the disease in these populations. The definition established in 1984 excluded 50–75% of infants and children with symptomatic HIV infection (Falloon, Eddy, Roper, & Pizzo, 1988). In 1987, the CDC modified the definition of AIDS for both adults and children. The modified definition is a better reflection of the spectrum of disease encountered in both groups. Table 5 (p.51) is a summary of the current surveillance definition of AIDS in children less than 13 years old.

CLASSIFICATION OF HIV INFECTION IN CHILDREN

The system used to classify HIV infection in infants and children was designed to include all who are infected with HIV, including those who are asymptomatic and those who have AIDS. The system is based on the CDC definitions of HIV infection and AIDS in children (see Table 6, p.52).

Class P-0, indeterminate infection, is used for infants less than 15 months old whose HIV status is unknown. Once the presence of HIV is established by diagnostic criteria, the infant should be reclassified.

Class P-1, asymptomatic infection, has three subclasses based on immune status: A, normal immune system; B, abnormal immune system; and C, immune function not tested. The abnormalities included in subclass B are hypo- or hypergammaglobulinemia, a reduction in the number of CD4 cells, a decrease in the ratio of CD4 to CD8 T cells, and absolute lymphopenia. Thus, class P-1-B indicates an asymptomatic child with an abnormal immune system.

Class P-2, symptomatic HIV infection, is divided into subclasses and categories on the basis of manifestations of illnesses and disorders.

Subclass A, nonspecific findings, is the assigned designation for the most common types of illnesses or problems seen. To be in this subclass, infants and children must have two or more signs or symptoms that have persisted for more than 2 months. Signs and symptoms are fever, failure to thrive, weight loss, hepatomegaly, splenomegaly, lymphadenopathy, parotitis, and diarrhea.

Subclass B, neurologic disease, includes the neurodevelopmental abnormalities that occur in an estimated 90% of infants and children who have HIV

Table 5
REVISED CDC DEFINITION OF AIDS

I. Without laboratory evidence of HIV infection, * a case of AIDS

- Does not have another cause of underlying immunodeficiency, and
- Has had one of a list of AIDS indicator diseases definitively diagnosed **

II. With laboratory evidence of HIV infection, a case of AIDS

- Has had one of a list of AIDS indicator diseases definitively diagnosed** or
- Has had one of a list of AIDS indicator diseases diagnosed presumptively*

III. With laboratory evidence against HIV infection (tests are negative), a case of AIDS

- Does not have another cause of underlying immunodeficiency, and
- Has had pneumocystiis pneumonia definitively diagnosed, or one of a list of AIDS indicator diseases definitively diagnosed and a CD4 count of $<400/mm^3$

*Tests not done or inconclusive. Includes seropositive children <15 months old with a seropositive mother and who have no other evidence of immunodeficiency or HIV infection.

**See chapter 1, "The CDC Definition of AIDS," sections I-B and II-A and B.

---

infection (Arpadi & Caspe, 1990). The most common abnormalities are acquired microcephaly, developmental delay, cognitive defects, and bilateral pyramidal tract signs. Developmental delays are failure to achieve developmental milestones or intellectual function. Pyramidal tract signs are motor abnormalities such as paresis, abnormal muscle tone, ataxia or gait disturbances, and pathologic reflexes.

Subclass C is lymphoid interstitial pneumonia, which occurs in 50% of infants and children who are infected with HIV (Arpadi & Caspe, 1990).

Subclass D includes the secondary infections that occur as a consequence of immunodeficiency. This subclass is further divided into categories that specify the nature of these infections. These are similar to the CDC classifications for AIDS in adults (see chapter 1). Category 1, opportunistic infections, includes PCP, cryptococcal infection, atypical or disseminated mycobacterial diseases, and candidiasis. Category 2, recurrent secondary bacterial infections, is the designation used when an infant or child has two or more secondary infections within 2 years. Sepsis, meningitis, abscesses in internal organs, pneumonia, and bone or joint infections may develop because of poor antibody response to common organisms such as *Streptococcus pneumoniae, Neisseria meningitidis, Hemophilus influenzae,* and *Salmonella enteritidis.* Category 3, severe recurrent viral infections, includes chronic and recurrent herpes stomatitis and disseminated or multidermatomal herpes zoster.

Subclass E, tumors, is subdivided into two categories. Category 1 includes primary central nervous system

> **Table 6**
> **CLASSIFICATION SYSTEM FOR HIV INFECTION IN CHILDREN**
>
> **Class P-0** Indeterminate Infection
>
> **Class P-1** Asymptomatic Infection
>
>   Subclass A   Normal immune system
>   Subclass B   Abnormal immune system
>   Subclass C   Immune function not determined
>
> **Class P-2** Symptomatic Infection
>
>   Subclass A   Nonspecific findings
>   Subclass B   Progressive neurological disease
>   Subclass C   Lymphoid interstitial pneumonia
>   Subclass D   Secondary infections
>
>   Category 1   Opportunistic infections
>   Category 2   Recurrent secondary bacterial infections
>   Category 3   Severe recurrent viral infections
>
>   Subclass E.   Secondary cancers
>
>   Category 1   Primary central nervous system lymphoma, Hodgkin's B-cell lymphoma, non-Hogkin's lymphoma, and Kaposi's sarcoma
>   Category 2   All other tumors potentially related to HIV infection
>
>   Subclass F.   Other diseases possibly related to HIV infection
>
> *Source: Arpadi & Caspe, 1990.*

lymphoma, Hodgkin's B-cell lymphoma, non-Hodgkin's lymphoma, and Kaposi's sarcoma (a rare tumor in infants and children). Category 2 includes all other tumors potentially related to HIV infection.

Subclass F includes all other diseases potentially related to HIV infection. Examples are cardiomyopathies, hematologic and renal disorders, and many of the skin disorders.

DIFFERENCES BETWEEN HIV DISEASE IN ADULTS AND IN INFANTS AND CHILDREN

HIV disease in infants and children differs from HIV disease in adults in many ways. The two major differences are the route of transmission and the size of the inoculum. Transmission of HIV in infants and children is primarily by the maternal route. Although the precise timing of infection is unknown, the size of the inoculum received by the fetus is thought to be large when transmission occurs in utero and much smaller if it occurs during birth (Clark, November 1992). The exact mechanism of transmission during delivery is not understood. The virus may be present in maternal blood that the infant swallows. The immature gastrointestinal system is unable to destroy the virus, and so the organism persists. The size of the inoculum the fetus receives in utero may be related to the effect of circulating maternal antibodies against HIV. High levels of antibody may reduce the size of the inoculum and thus may provide the fetus some protection. All these situations may help explain why only 20–35% of infants born to HIV-infected women are infected with the virus (Bernstein et al., 1989; Clark, November 1992; Novello et al., 1989).

A larger inoculum may also cause increased damage to the growing brain of the fetus, which may result in chronic encephalopathy after birth. Loss of developmental milestones and mental and motor retardation may be indications of this. However, these conditions are also affected by problems associated with drug abuse and poor nutrition in the mother, so determining the exact cause may be difficult.

A defective humoral immune system leads to other differences in HIV disease in infants and children. Because of the inability to mobilize effective antibodies, recurrent, severe bacterial infections and lung diseases develop. Infections due to bacteria are more common in infants and children, whereas opportunistic infections due to other kinds of microorganisms are more common in adults.

Other differences are the length of incubation and the shorter time between the symptomatic phase and death. HIV disease progresses more rapidly in infants and children than in adults. In most infants, signs and symptoms of advanced infection develop in the first 18 months of life (Connor, 1991).

Pulmonary lymphocytic hyperplasia and lymphoid interstitial pneumonia are more progressive, severe, and common in children than in adults. Brain lymphomas are common in children, but Kaposi's sarcoma is not. Finally, laboratory parameters are different. The normal CD4 count in children may be as high as 3,500 cells/mm^3. A decrease to 1,500 cells/mm^3 indicates severe immunosuppression. Therefore, the CD4 count is higher in children than in adults when signs and symptoms of AIDS become evident. Children also have less of a reversal in the ratio of CD4 to CD8 T cells and have elevated levels of lactic dehydrogenase (Bernstein et al., 1989; Novello et al., 1989).

CLINICAL MANIFESTATIONS OF HIV DISEASE IN INFANTS AND CHILDREN

In some cases, progressive encephalopathy is the only manifestation of HIV infection acquired in utero or at birth. The abnormality develops slowly and gradually and worsens proportionately as the level of immunodeficiency increases. Subacute encephalopathy causes a gradual decrease in alertness, increasing apathy, gradual inability to play, and, finally, loss of interest in the surrounding environment. Older children may also have developmental delays or a deterioration in motor skills and intellectual functioning.

The encephalopathy is often accompanied by neurologic abnormalities, which result in generalized muscle weakness and an ataxic gait. Paresis, abnormal tone, and hypotonia with bilateral pathologic reflexes may be observed early in the course of the abnormality. Later, spastic quadriparesis and pseudobulbar palsy may develop. Seizures are rare unless the child has a febrile illness or other central nervous system problems, such as tumors or brain lesions.

Because HIV infection prevents development of immunologic memory in infants and children, bacterial infections are recurrent and are a major problem. In children, serious bacterial infections such as meningitis, pneumonia, sepsis, abscesses, and cellulitis are often the first manifestation of AIDS. The most common pathogens are *S. pneumoniae*, *H. influenzae*, *Staphylococcus aureus*, *Staphylococcus epidermidis*, and *Salmonella* species. These infections affect the skin, nose, throat, ears, and lungs. Infections of the lungs, gastrointestinal tract, central nervous system,

Table 7
CLINICAL MANIFESTATION OF HIV INFECTION IN CHILDREN

Common Findings

- Low birth weight
- Failure to thrive
- Weight loss
- Fevers
- Malaise
- Lymphadenopathy
- Hepatosplenomegaly
- Recurrent upper respiratory infections (otitis, sinusitis, pneumonias)
- Digital clubbing
- Eczema or other skin rashes
- Persistent thrush and *Candida* diaper infections
- Chronic or recurrent diarrhea
- Developmental delay
- Encephalopathy
- Microencephalopathy
- Neurologic manifestations
- Recurrent nonrespiratory bacterial and viral infections

Less Common Findings

- Opportunistic infections
- Hepatitis
- Cardiomyopathy
- Nephropathy
- Parotitis or salivary gland enlargement
- HIV dysmorphology and embryopathy
- Thrombocytopenia
- Kaposi's sarcoma
- B-cell lymphoma

Source: Bernstein et al., 1989; Wishon & Gee, 1988; Wiznia & Rubinstein, 1988.

hemopoietic system, and other organs are a major cause of morbidity and mortality.

Many of the clinical manifestations of HIV disease in infants and children are similar to those in adults (Table 7). The physical abnormality seen most often is failure to thrive. Recurrent infections are common. Many children have chronic and recurrent episodes of diarrhea, otitis media, pneumonia, bacterial sepsis, persistent thrush, and rashes. Physical examination may show thrush, lymphadenopathy, and perineal rashes. Other physical signs include those that indicate systemic disease, such as fever or growth and neurologic abnormalities. Figure 10 (p.55) shows the ratio of the incidence rate of signs and symptoms of HIV infection in pre-AIDS HIV-infected and uninfected children born to infected mothers.

DIAGNOSTIC EVALUATION AND MEDICAL MANAGEMENT

The specific tests used to diagnose and evaluate HIV disease in infants and children are the same as those used in adults. General tests include CBC and differential, platelet count, chemistry panel, enumer-

CHAPTER 5 —
HIV DISEASE IN INFANTS, CHILDREN, AND ADOLESCENTS

Figure 10
SIGNS AND SYMPTOMS ASSOCIATED WITH HIV INFECTION IN CHILDREN

Ratio of the incidence rate in pre-AIDS HIV-infected and uninfected children born to infected mothers

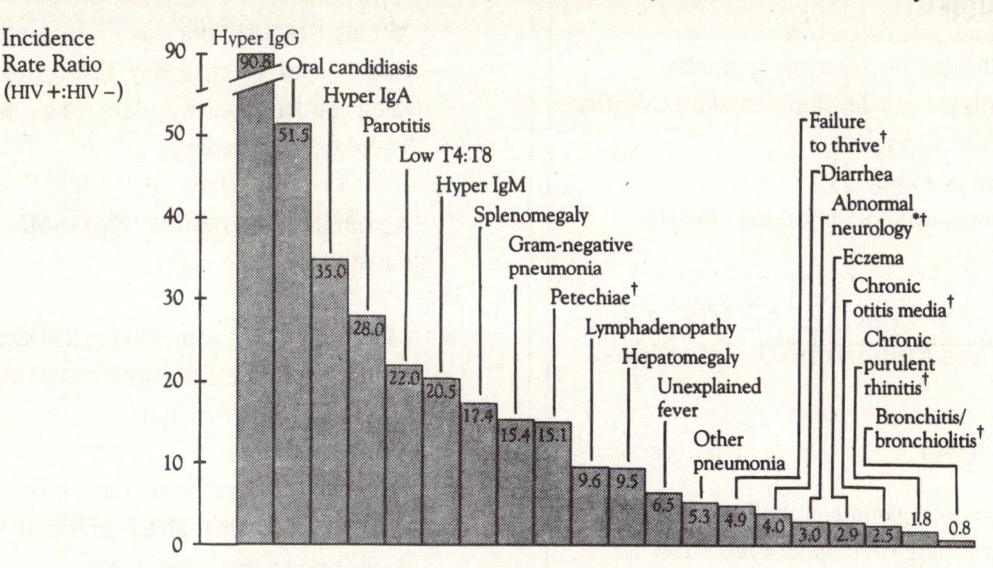

Incidence Rate Ratio (HIV +:HIV −)

Sign/Symptom	Ratio
Hyper IgG	90.8
Oral candidiasis	51.5
Hyper IgA	35.0
Parotitis	28.0
Low T4:T8	22.0
Hyper IgM	20.5
Splenomegaly	17.4
Gram-negative pneumonia	15.4
Petechiae[†]	15.1
Lymphadenopathy	9.6
Hepatomegaly	9.5
Unexplained fever	6.5
Other pneumonia	5.3
Failure to thrive[†]	4.9
Diarrhea	4.0
Abnormal neurology[*†]	3.0
Eczema	2.9
Chronic otitis media[†]	2.5
Chronic purulent rhinitis[†]	1.8
Bronchitis/bronchiolitis[†]	0.8

[*]Abnormal neurology other than encephalopathy: abnormal reflexes or gait, seizures, paresis
[†]Difference between rates in HIV + and HIV − children not significant at P = 0.01

Source: Portions of the publication, "AIDS Clinical Care" are reprinted by permission. ACC (c) 3:24, 3:32. Massachusetts Medical Society. All rights reserved.

---

ation of T-cell subsets, quantitative determination of levels of immunoglobulins, chest radiograph, and CT scan of the head. Specific tests depend on the current signs and symptoms, the potential system or organ involved, or the suspected causative agent of the current disorder.

The three types of treatment of HIV disease in infants and children are general supportive therapy, prevention and treatment of infections, and support of the existing immune function.

Supportive therapy includes nutritional support; treatment of tumors, organ failure, and chronic pain; psychosocial support; and education of the patient and the patient's family and significant others.

Treatments specific for HIV disease in children lag behind those for adults, partly because of the slow detection of the disease in children. General management of opportunistic infections in children with HIV disease is summarized in Table 8 (p.56).

Prevention of opportunistic infections is difficult because there is no specific intervention for the underlying immunodeficiency. Most preventive treatment has been aimed at reducing these infections and hospitalizations and delaying the progression of HIV disease. The primary intervention for reducing opportunistic infections has been immunosupportive therapy, which is discussed later in this chapter.

The major thrust of medical intervention is treatment of existing opportunistic infections and prophylactic therapy. For the most part, treatment of any infection is similar to that used in adults. The therapy may not be dramatic and frequently is designed to improve quality of life (Table 9, p. 57–59).

> **Table 8**
> **GENERAL MANAGEMENT OF HIV-INFECTED CHILDREN**
>
> **General Support**
>
> > A multidisciplinary team approach
> > Neurologic and developmental interventions
> > Nutritional support
> > Patient advocacy
> > Immunization for childhood diseases
>
> **Therapy and Prophylaxis for HIV-Related Problems and Opportunistic Infections**
>
> > Immunotherapy
> >
> > > Intravenous gamma globulin
> > > Other biological response modifiers
> >
> > Antiviral Chemotherapy and Chemoprophylaxis
> >
> > > Zidovudine
> > > Other drugs proved effective by research
>
> **Prevention**
>
> > Education that targets young children and adolescents
> > Risk reduction for uninfected women of childbearing age
> > Family planning and counseling for HIV-infected women
>
> *Source:* Adapted from Bernstein et al., 1989.

Guidelines for prophylaxis against PCP have recently been established by the CDC (1991b). Pneumocystis pneumonia is the most common serious HIV-related opportunistic infection among children, so primary prophylaxis makes sense. Recommendations and information on when to start PCP prophylaxis in children are given in Figure 11 (p.60). The drug regimens for children are as follows (CDC, 1991b):

1. Recommended regimen (infants at least 1 month old): Trimethoprim/sulfamethoxazole (TMP-SMX) 150 mg TMP/m^2 per day with 750 mg SMX/m^2 per day given orally in divided doses twice a day three times each week on consecutive days (e.g., Monday, Tuesday, Wednesday)

2. Acceptable alternative TMP-SMX dosage schedules:

   - 150 mg TMP/m^2 with 750 mg SMX/m^2 given orally as a single daily dose three times each week on consecutive days

   - 150 mg TMP/m^2 per day with 750 mg SMX/m^2 per day given orally in divided doses twice a day 7 days/week

   - 150 mg TMP/m^2 per day with 750 mg SMX/m^2 per day given orally in divided doses twice a day three times each week on alternate days (e.g., Monday, Wednesday, Friday)

3. Alternative regimens if TMP-SMX not tolerated:

   - Dapsone (children at least 1 month old): 1 mg/kg (not to exceed 100 mg) given orally once daily

   - Aerosolized pentamidine (children at least 5 years old): 300 mg given via Respirgard II inhaler monthly

   - If neither dapsone nor aerosolized pentamidine is tolerated, some clinicians use intravenous pentamidine (4 mg/kg) given every 2 or 4 weeks

Table 9
TREATMENT OF INFECTIONS IN CHILDREN WITH HIV DISEASE

Pathogen	Manifestation	Drug(s)	Dosage	Side Effects
Pneumocystis carinii	Pneumonia	Trimethoprim (TMP) and	20 mg/kg per day divided into four doses	Nausea, vomiting, diarrhea, fever, rash leukopenia, neutropenia, anemia
		Sulfamethoxazole (SMX)	100 mg/kg per day divided into four doses given intravenously or orally for 2–3 weeks	
		Pentamidine	4 mg/kg once a day intravenously or intramuscularly* for 2–3 weeks	Hypoglycemia, neutropenia, abscesses at injection site
		TMP and SMX for prophylaxis	5 mg and 25 mg divided into two equal doses given 3 days each week	
Toxoplasma gondii	Brain abscesses Bone marrow infections	Sulfadiazine and	120 mg/kg per day divided into four doses given orally	Rash, nausea, vomiting, diarrhea
		Pyrimethamine and	2 mg/kg per day divided into two doses given orally for 3 days and then 1 mg/kg per day, with a maximum of 25 mg once a day	Bone marrow suppression
		Folinic acid	5–10 mg/day	
Cryptosporidium	Diarrhea	None to date	Supportive therapy	

* Intramuscular route rarely used because of complications of abscesses

Table 9
TREATMENT OF INFECTIONS IN CHILDREN WITH HIV DISEASE
(Continued)

Pathogen	Manifestation	Drug(s)	Dosage	Side Effects
Cryptococcus neoformans	Meningitis, fungemia, and pneumonia	Amphotericin B	1 mg/kg intravenously daily	Fevers, chills, renal toxic effects, leukopenia, neutropenia, hypokalemia, decreased levels of magnesium and phosphate
		5-Flucytosine	150 mg/kg per day orally divided into four doses	Rash, nausea, vomiting
Candida	Thrush, esophagitis, perineal infections	Nystatin liquid	0.6 ml swabbed in mouth or as a swish and swallow four to five times each day	Diarrhea
		Nystatin suppository	Dissolved in mouth one to five times each day	
		Clotrimazole troche	10 mg dissolved in the mouth one to five times each day	
		Ketoconazole (for severe thrush or esophagitis)	5–10 mg/kg orally once a day	Abnormal liver function tests
		Clotrimazole or nystatin creams	Applied to rash area	
Mycobacterium avium-intracellulare	Pneumonia, central nervous system, disseminated	No standard treatment		

Table 9
TREATMENT OF INFECTIONS IN CHILDREN
(Continued)

Pathogen	Syndrome	Drug(s)	Dosage	Side Effects
Mycobacterium tuberculosis	Pulmonary, central nervous system, disseminated	Isoniazid (INH)	10–20 mg/kg per day orally	Liver function abnormalities, rash
		Rifampin	10–20 mg/kg per day orally not to exceed 600 mg/day Use with INH for 9–12 months	Rash, liver function abnormalities, neutropenia
		Pyrazinamide	20–30 mg/kg per day for 2 months	
	Positive skin tests	INH prophylaxis	10–20 mg/kg per day for 1 year	
Cytomegalovirus	Chorioretinitis	Ganciclovir	5 mg/kg/ twice a day for 2 weeks, then 5 mg/kg per day for indefinite period	Neutropenia, anemia, development of resistance
	Pneumonitis, hepatitis, colitis, esophagitis, encephalitis, disseminated	No treatment, although some may use ganciclovir		
Herpes simplex virus	Stomatitis, perianal ulcers	Acyclovir	750 mg/m^2 per day intravenously or orally divided into four to five doses	Renal toxic effects
Varicella-zoster virus	Primary chickenpox, local or disseminated	Acyclovir	1500 mg/m^2 per day intravenously divided into four doses	Renal toxic effects

Figure 11
RECOMMENDATIONS FOR PCP PROPHYLAXIS IN CHILDREN

Recommendations are for children >1 month old who are HIV infected, HIV seropositive, or <12 months old and born to an HIV-infected mother.

A CD4+ count and CD4+% should be obtained for each child. Use test results and child's age as criteria for starting PCP prophylaxis.

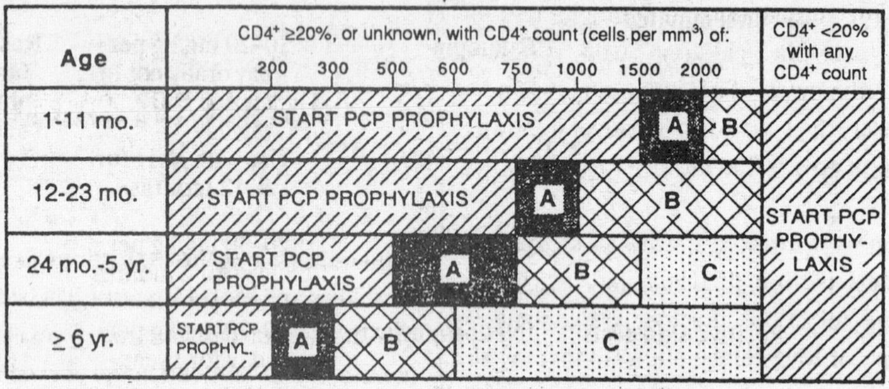

Age	CD4+ ≥20%, or unknown, with CD4+ count (cells per mm³) of: 200 300 500 600 750 1000 1500 2000	CD4+ <20% with any CD4+ count
1-11 mo.	START PCP PROPHYLAXIS ... A > B	START PCP PROPHYLAXIS
12-23 mo.	START PCP PROPHYLAXIS ... A ... B	
24 mo.-5 yr.	START PCP PROPHYLAXIS ... A ... B ... C	
≥ 6 yr.	START PCP PROPHYL. ... A ... B ... C	

A: No prophylaxis recommended at this time: recheck CD4+ count in 1 month.
B: No prophylaxis recommended at this time: recheck CD4+ count at least every 3-4 months.
C: No prophylaxis recommended at this time: recheck CD4+ count at least every 6 months.

Recommended regimen for PCP prophylaxis

Trimethoprim/sulfamethoxazole (TMP-SMX) 150 mg TMP/M²/day with 750 mg SMX/M²/day given orally in divided doses twice a day, 3 times per week, on consecutive days (e.g., Monday-Tuesday-Wednesday). When starting TMP-SMX prophylaxis:

- Obtain baseline CBC, differential count, platelet count.
- Monitor CBC, differential count, platelet count monthly.
- Monitor CD4+ count at least every three months.

Note: PCP=Pneumocystis Carinii Pneumonia. Any child who has had an episode of PCP should be started on PCP prophylaxis regardless of age or CD4+ count.

Source: Centers for Disease Control, 1991a.

Zidovudine and intravenous immunoglobulin are used for immunosupportive therapy. Zidovudine has recently been approved by the Food and Drug Administration (FDA) for treatment of AIDS or signs and symptoms of advanced HIV disease in young children. Until now, the drug had been approved only for use in children more than 13 years old. The new approval allows prescription of zidovudine for children at least 3 months old. The recommended dose for young children is 180 mg/m² (body surface) every 6 hr by mouth. The maximum dose should not exceed 200 mg every 6 hr. The drug is available in 100-mg capsules and as a strawberry-flavored syrup of 50 mg/5 ml. Studies are continuing to determine the minimum dose required each day (Katzin, 1990). Side effects of zidovudine in children are the same as in adults. These include anemia, neutropenia, nausea, vomiting, diarrhea, and lethargy (Katzin, 1990).

Intravenous immunoglobulin therapy was initially used to decrease the prevalence of bacterial infections and reduce the number of hospital admissions. Because no control studies were done to evaluate the effectiveness of this therapy for these conditions, it still lacks firm support (Falloon et al., 1988). Preventive therapy with intravenous immunoglobulin is based on its use in children with primary hypogammaglobulinemias. The immunoglobulin is administered every 2–3 weeks over several hours. The most common dose is 200 mg/kg (Yap, 1990).

Nutritional support is directed toward managing the effects of anorexia, chronic diarrhea, malabsorption, and chronic oral infections. Lactose intolerance is frequent because of long-term antibiotic therapy or an inability to digest lactose. Lactose-free formulas such as Soylac and Isocal can be used for children with lactose intolerance. Vitamin and mineral supplements may also be needed, along with nutritional guidance, to ensure that the child is receiving double the recommended daily allowances (Klug, 1986).

Diarrhea is the most common cause of dehydration and loss of electrolytes. Infants need to be monitored especially closely when they have diarrhea or are vomiting. Adequate hydration must be maintained. Solutions high in glucose and electrolytes should be used to supplement other food or liquid intake (Wishon & Gee, 1988).

The lesions of thrush and oral herpes infections are difficult to manage. They may interfere with an infant's ability to suck or a child's ability to chew food. Regular use of prescribed antithrush medications, even in the absence of thrush, will help control and prevent this infection. A soft or bland diet is often better tolerated than a regular diet is. Cold foods may decrease mouth pain, whereas hot foods may increase it. Use of a straw, when possible, may also alleviate pain caused by some foods and beverages (Klug, 1986).

Little information is available on appropriate treatments for tumors, organ failure, and chronic pain. Children with tumors that may respond to therapy should be referred to a pediatric hematologist/oncologist. Treatment would is similar to that used in immunocompetent children.

IMMUNIZATIONS

Immunization against infectious diseases with high morbidity and mortality rates has been a major goal of child health care for many years. However, immunization of immunocompromised children is still controversial. One question is whether immunizations might weaken the immune system more. Live viruses in some vaccines might undergo enhanced replication and thus pose a potentially serious health threat to immunocompromised children. Other concerns center on whether an immune system that is depressed or altered will react to exposure to antigens.

The CDC and WHO have established recommendations (Table 10, p.63) for immunizations that are based on the severity of immunosuppression (CDC, 1986c). Children who are asymptomatic or who are not immunocompromised should receive live virus and bacterial vaccines. The adverse reaction to attenuated live measles vaccine in severely ill children with HIV disease is considered preferable to the high mortality associated with measles in these children.

PSYCHOSOCIAL ISSUES

Providing care for infants and children who have HIV disease is an enormous problem. Many of the children in New York and New Jersey who have the disease are permanent patients in hospitals because their families cannot care for them and foster care is not available. These children will not develop emotional and social skills normally learned in the family environment unless nurses and other health care providers are aware of the socialization needs of these patients (Task Force on Pediatric AIDS, 1989).

In many families, the stages of coping with HIV disease are similar to the stages of coping with death and dying described by Kubler-Ross (1969). Parents may experience isolation from family and friends. Stress from financial burdens may increase the sense of uncertainty and inadequacy. Loss of control, lack of confidence in parenting abilities, anxiety about the child's medical condition, and guilt may increase stress and decrease coping. These issues must be recognized and interventions planned.

Infants and children with HIV disease place an additional burden on those parents who lack appropriate parenting knowledge and skills. Placing their own needs first, drug users may neglect their children in search of drugs. The combination of drug use and poor parenting increases the risks for infants and children, who are unable to care for themselves.

In some situations, the mother's own HIV disease causes more problems. Her health may interfere with her ability to provide adequate physical and emotional support to the infected child and to any other children in the family. These same health problems may also affect her relationship with a spouse or sexual partner, and thus the family's stability. Frequently, the mother is dealing not only with her own death and dying issues but also with those of her spouse and her children.

Individual and family emotional problems can be managed through counseling and AIDS support groups. Financial and care provider support may also be available through various community organizations. Negotiating the maze of governmental agencies can make a parent's sense of helplessness worse and increase frustration and anger toward the child, the disease, and society. In order to alleviate these frustrations, a social worker's assistance should be provided.

Emotional and social problems may be related to a lack of day care centers and schools that willingly accept infants or children who have HIV disease. These issues may need to be dealt with on a community rather than an individual level. Inadequate or unavailable child support systems, however, can affect the parents' ability to work and earn an income.

An atmosphere of fear and rejection forces many parents to hide the child's true diagnosis. They describe the illness as cancer or some other terminal illness. Families that are open about the diagnosis sometimes are excluded from social activities and ostracized, as friends withdraw because of fear. Helping parents decide whom to tell and when can help alleviate some of their social isolation and stigmatization (Wishon & Gee, 1988).

Finally, the child's coping patterns depend on cognitive development and the social network. Adverse reactions by others can increase the child's anger and frustration and lead to isolation or lack of appropriate socialization. The family's ability to care for the child and the child's ability to attend school are related to community atmosphere and the condition of the child. Hospital admissions interrupt family, school, and social activities and increase isolation. Health care providers should encourage children who have HIV disease to socialize and attend as many functions as possible.

Table 10
SUMMARY OF RECOMMENDATIONS FOR IMMUNIZATION OF CHILDREN WITH HIV INFECTION

Vaccine	Symptomatic Infection	Asymptomatic Infection	Not Known To Be Infected	Resides in Household with Person with AIDS	Age to Vaccinate
Measles, mumps, rubella (MMR)	Yes	Yes**	Yes**	Yes	15 months
Oral polio * (OPV)	No	No	Yes	No	2, 4, and 6 months
Bacille Calmette-Guerin (BCG)	No	No	No	No	
Inactivated polio (IPV)	Yes**	Yes	Yes**	Yes	2, 4, and 6 months
Hemophilus influenzae type B (HIB)	Yes**	Yes**	Yes**		18 months
Diphtheria, tetanus, pertussis (DTP)	Yes**	Yes**	Yes		2, 4, and 6 months
Pneumococcal vaccine (PV)	Yes	Yes	Yes	Yes	After 2 years of age
Inactivated influenza virus	Yes	Yes		Yes	After 6 months of age and then yearly

* Live vaccines and live bacterial vaccines

**Immunization is recommended according to the U.S. Public Health Advisory Committee on Immunization Practice.

Source: Adapted from Lewis & Thomson, 1989. See also Centers for Disease Control, 1989c.

EDUCATION OF CHILDREN AND PARENTS

Many issues affect transmission of HIV in children. Two of the most important are education and poverty. Communities must address the issues of poverty that lead to drug abuse and pregnancy. Educators must determine the needs of the community and the individual. Educational programs should be developed to fight poverty and drug abuse and promote behavioral changes that will eliminate these problems and the spread of HIV infection.

Educational efforts should be directed to families directly affected by HIV disease and to the community at large. Both groups need to understand the disease process and the risk of infection in order to protect themselves, other family members, and the child. Decisions about protection from infection should be made by weighing risks against benefits. Families and care providers should be educated about child care, nutrition, and any services available to assist with care (Mendez, 1990).

Children should also be the focus of education and preventive measures. As HIV disease becomes more widespread in the heterosexual population, programs geared toward prevention should begin at an early age. Children with HIV disease should be informed about the disease process and about what is happening to them. The amount of information given will depend on their level of understanding and cognitive development.

Community education is also important in preventing transmission of the virus and stigmatization of infected persons. Communities should have ongoing programs that provide up-to-date, accurate information about transmission of HIV and ways to prevent it. These should include programs that teach and reinforce behavioral changes that will prevent the spread of the virus.

Finally, HIV disease in children can be prevented. Women of childbearing age must abstain from drug use and sexual contacts that increase their risk for HIV infection. Women who are already infected should be counseled about the risks of transmitting HIV to their fetus if they become pregnant and the effect the disease may have on pregnant women.

NURSING CARE

Nursing care for infants and children with HIV disease is similar to that for adults. Infection control procedures (CDC, 1985a) should be followed for both hospitalized children and those treated at home. Nursing care should be supportive and nonjudgmental. Consideration should be given to the developmental, nutritional, respiratory, hematologic, and psychosocial needs of the child and to the psychosocial needs of the child's care providers.

Nursing assessment is important both in the hospital and in the home setting (Berry, 1988). The initial and ongoing assessments provide a basis for the development of an individualized care plan. Whenever possible, the child and the child's family or care providers should be involved in developing the plan of care. Nursing diagnoses may include any of the following:

- Alteration in
    nutrition
    respiratory and/or bowel function
    growth and development
    comfort
    parenting
    coping (family and/or child)

- Potential for
    injury

infection
bleeding
social isolation related to
    fatigue
    ignorance
    deterioration
    physical status

- Disturbance in self-concept due to
  disease process
  social stigma

- Knowledge deficits relating to
  disease process,
  infection control
  nutrition
  developmental milestones
  available resources
  provision of care

HIV DISEASE IN ADOLESCENTS

Epidemiology and Demographics

By the end of 1988, AIDS had been diagnosed in 421 adolescents 13–19 years old. More than half the adolescents who have HIV disease are members of minority groups. The male-to-female ratio is 3:1 in New York and 7:1 in other parts of the United States (Nicholas, Sondheimer, Willoughby, Yaffe, & Katz, 1989).

Most persons with AIDS who were in their early 20s when the syndrome was diagnosed were probably infected with HIV when they were teenagers. Early in the epidemic, teenagers were infected by means of HIV-contaminated blood products. Today, adolescents acquire HIV primarily through sexual contact and the sharing of needles and syringes. Another factor that must be considered in this age group is the possibility of pregnancy among sexually active adolescent girls (Novello et al., 1989).

Adolescents are at increased risk for HIV disease because of their ignorance about the disease, their not-me attitude, and their tendency to deny their mortality (Bernstein et al., 1989). Adolescent sexual encounters (homosexual or heterosexual) are often experimental, inexperienced, random, spontaneous, anonymous, and promiscuous. Use of drugs and alcohol further increases the risk. These substances lower inhibitions and lead to more random and spontaneous sexual encounters and increased promiscuity. In those who are addicted, the need for money to buy drugs or alcohol can lead to prostitution. The additional problems of disrupted homes and families and runaways, which frequently lead to drug abuse, prostitution, and sexual promiscuity, will also affect the increase of HIV infection in adolescents.

Although sexual activity varies by race, age, sex, ethnic background, and socioeconomic characteristics, evidence indicates that nowadays sexual activity begins at an earlier age and increases steadily during adolescence. One study found that 0.2% of randomly selected college students in the United States were seropositive for HIV at the end of 1988 (Bernstein et al., 1989). This percentage is low, but it is expected that the number of cases of HIV disease among teenagers and young adults will continue to increase.

Serologic Testing and Diagnosis

Serologic testing and diagnosis of HIV disease are the same for adolescents and adults. In order to provide early detection of the disease and intervention, tests for antibodies to HIV should be considered for teenagers who use drugs and are sexually active. Testing should include counseling that ensures confidentiality. Consent for testing may be a problem if permission from a parent or conservator is required.

Nurses involved in counseling and testing should be aware of laws and policies pertaining to testing of teenagers.

Counseling should include (1) evaluation of the teenager's risk behaviors, knowledge about HIV disease, emotional response, and support systems and (2) information on follow-up medical care and services. Adolescents who are seronegative should receive information on how to prevent HIV infection. Those who are seropositive should be counseled on how to prevent transmission, about issues associated with pregnancy, and about local resources.

Assessment and Treatment

Assessment of any teenager is a challenge. Establishing rapport frequently is difficult, especially on first-time visits. Health care providers can put a teenager at ease by being direct yet sensitive to personal and confidentiality issues. They should begin by explaining why HIV disease in a matter of concern for teenagers and then ask questions and give advice. Noting the relation of the disease to adult issues may encourage rapport.

Adolescents should be questioned about risk behaviors for HIV disease every time they seek medical care for any problem, especially sexually transmitted diseases. Assessment should include routine laboratory and radiologic tests (see chapter 7). Tests to detect sexually transmitted diseases and hepatitis B should be part of all evaluations. If the teenager has anemia or leukopenia, additional tests should be done to determine the cause and enable early intervention (Bernstein et al., 1989).

Medical management of HIV infection, opportunistic infections, and tumors in adolescents is the same as that used in adults. See chapter 7 for details.

Psychosocial Issues

Many of the psychosocial issues of adolescents who have HIV disease are directly related to image and self-concept and the stigma of the disease. Health care providers should be aware of these issues. Teenagers who have HIV disease should be encouraged to talk about how the disease affects their lives.

Fear, rejection, and decreasing physical stamina may result in social isolation and withdrawal. Teenagers should be encouraged to maintain social contacts and, at the same time, attempt to reduce their friends' fears of contagion. Care providers should provide a listening ear, minimize giving advice, and be nonjudgmental when interacting with an adolescent.

Disenfranchised adolescents may be angry at family members or relatives over abandonment issues. Reconciliation of family and friends should be considered and attempted if possible. When this is not possible, health care providers can help the teenager develop other support systems to cope with the disease and foster inclusion rather than abandonment.

Those teenagers who live with family members or have been reconciled may feel guilty and ashamed for having HIV disease. They may feel that they have let down the family or siblings. Health care providers must be ready to listen to these concerns and fears and be safe persons with whom anger may be ventilated. Reestablishment of self-worth may be slow, but it is an essential ingredient in the teenager's ability to cope with the consequences of HIV disease.

Education

Teaching adolescents about HIV disease is difficult. One reason is the characteristics of this age group. Teenagers frequently view themselves as invincible, and they are risk takers. Another reason is society's ambivalence about drugs and sexually explicit educational programs. Little research has been done on

CHAPTER 5 —
HIV DISEASE IN INFANTS, CHILDREN, AND ADOLESCENTS

sexual behavior and drug and alcohol use in adolescents, and no studies have been done on the effectiveness of behavior-modification programs for teenagers.

Educational programs about HIV disease must be provided, even though valid evidence about what will be effective is not available. These programs should stress that AIDS is a matter of life and death for adolescents and young adults. To promote honest communication between adults and teenagers, educators, health practitioners, and parents need to be open and accepting. Parents and health care providers should encourage teenagers to become knowledgeable about the disease and how HIV is transmitted and prevented. They should offer to answer any question a teenager may have and should consider no question too trivial to answer. If an adult cannot answer a question, he or she should direct the teenager to someone who can. Teenagers should be encouraged to practice sexual abstinence and not use drugs and alcohol. Adolescents who are sexually active should be encouraged to use latex condoms and spermicidal agents with nonoxynol-9.

The next chapter discusses drugs and therapies being used or developed to treat HIV disease.

EXAM QUESTIONS

Chapter 5

Questions 28 - 43

28. Antibodies produced by an infant cannot be distinguished from antibodies received from the mother for approximately how many months after birth?

    a. 12 months
    b. 18 months ✓
    c. 21 months
    d. 24 months

29. What are the reasons adolescents are at increased risk for HIV infection?

    a. Denial of mortality, inexperience, planned sex, multiple partners
    b. Denial of mortality, experimentation, unsafe sex, single partner
    c. Spontaneity, experimentation, unsafe sex, single partner
    d. Denial of mortality, inexperience, spontaneity, experimentation ✓

30. Which of the following vaccines should asymptomatic HIV-infected children receive?

    a. Bacille Calmette-Guerin
    b. Measles, mumps, rubella ✓
    c. Hepatitis B
    d. Oral polio

31. Currently, the number of infants and children in the United States infected with HIV may be more than:

    a. 20,000 ✓
    b. 40,000
    c. 60,000
    d. 80,000

32. What are the three types of medical treatment of HIV disease in infants and children?

    a. Supportive therapy, prevention and treatment of infections, support of existing immune function ✓
    b. Supportive therapy, family education, prevention of infections
    c. Treatment of infections, support of existing immune function, psychologic therapy
    d. Psychologic therapy, social services, treatment of infections

33. The size of the inoculum, encephalopathy, and recurrent bacterial infections are a few of the differences in HIV infection in which of the following groups?

    a. Infants and children ✓
    b. Children and adolescents
    c. Children and adults
    d. Adolescents and adults

34. What disease or disorder do failure to thrive, lymphadenopathy, hepatosplenomegaly, chronic diarrhea, and recurrent bacterial infections in children suggest?

    a. AIDS
    b. Cystic fibrosis
    c. HIV infection
    d. Congenital immunodeficiency

35. Many of the psychosocial issues of HIV-infected adolescents are directly related to image and self-concept and:

    a. Medical management of the disease
    b. The stigma of the disease
    c. Education
    d. Anger

36. What are the three criteria used to diagnose HIV infection in children more than 15 months old?

    a. Symptomatic infection, antibodies to HIV, and lymphadenopathy
    b. HIV antigen, antibodies to HIV, and signs and symptoms of infection
    c. HIV antigen, CDC-defined AIDS, and progressive neurologic disease
    d. Antibodies to HIV, HIV in blood or tissues, symptoms of CDC-defined AIDS

37. Two reasons HIV disease is becoming more prevalent in the United States are:

    a. Drug abuse and poverty
    b. Drug use and sex
    c. Lack of education and money
    d. Poverty and fear

38. At what age do infants begin to develop their own immunoglobulins or antibodies?

    a. 1–3 months
    b. 4–6 months
    c. 9–12 months
    d. 18–21 months

39. Which of the following is a drug used to treat HIV disease in children?

    a. Zidovudine
    b. Alpha-interferon
    c. Acyclovir
    d. Peptide T

40. What is the most common clinical manifestation of perinatal HIV infection?

    a. Neurodevelopmental deficits
    b. Bacterial infection
    c. Failure to thrive
    d. Chronic diarrhea

41. What are the two most serious issues affecting transmission of HIV in children?

    a. Options besides drug abuse and pregnancy
    b. Education of children and adults
    c. Drug abuse and police protection
    d. Education and poverty

42. What is one way to put teenagers at ease and obtain information about risk factors?

    a. Ask general impersonal questions
    b. Ask questions about sex last
    c. Be direct yet sensitive
    d. Be brisk and authoritative

43. A common nutritional problem in children with HIV disease is:

   a. Weight gain
   b. Lactose intolerance
   c. Hyperglycemia
   d. Food allergies

CHAPTER 6

TREATMENT OF HIV DISEASE

CHAPTER OBJECTIVE

After studying this chapter, the reader will be able to discuss drug and nondrug therapies proposed, being studied, and being used to treat HIV disease.

LEARNING OBJECTIVES

After studying this chapter, the reader should be able to

1. Describe the process by which the FDA approves drugs and establishes indications for treatment with a drug.

2. Specify one of the drugs approved by the FDA for use against HIV and describe its side effects.

3. Name the potential drug for treatment of HIV disease that is effective against respiratory syncytial virus infections.

4. Name the antiviral and anti-HIV drug that was originally used as an antiparasitic drug in Africa.

5. Name the two compounds similar to zidovudine that have been approved for treatment of HIV infection.

6. Name two drugs currently being studied as virus-receptor inhibitors for HIV infection.

INTRODUCTION

The identification, isolation, and characterization of the causative agent of AIDS occurred very quickly. Extensive knowledge of the structure, replication, and epidemiology of HIV has led to the licensing of three drugs for treatment of HIV disease. Many other drugs are under study, and numerous additional strategies and diverse targets of attack have been suggested (Mildvan & Richman, 1989; Richman, 1988a). Figure 12 (p.72) shows the life cycle of HIV, possible points of therapeutic intervention, and examples of agents proposed to inhibit replication of HIV type 1.

Characterization of virus-specific targets has provided multiple possibilities for the design of drugs that inhibit HIV. For optimal results, drugs used to treat HIV disease must (1) cross the blood-brain barrier and penetrate the cerebrospinal fluid, (2) be fea-

Figure 12
THE LIFE CYCLE OF HIV TYPE I

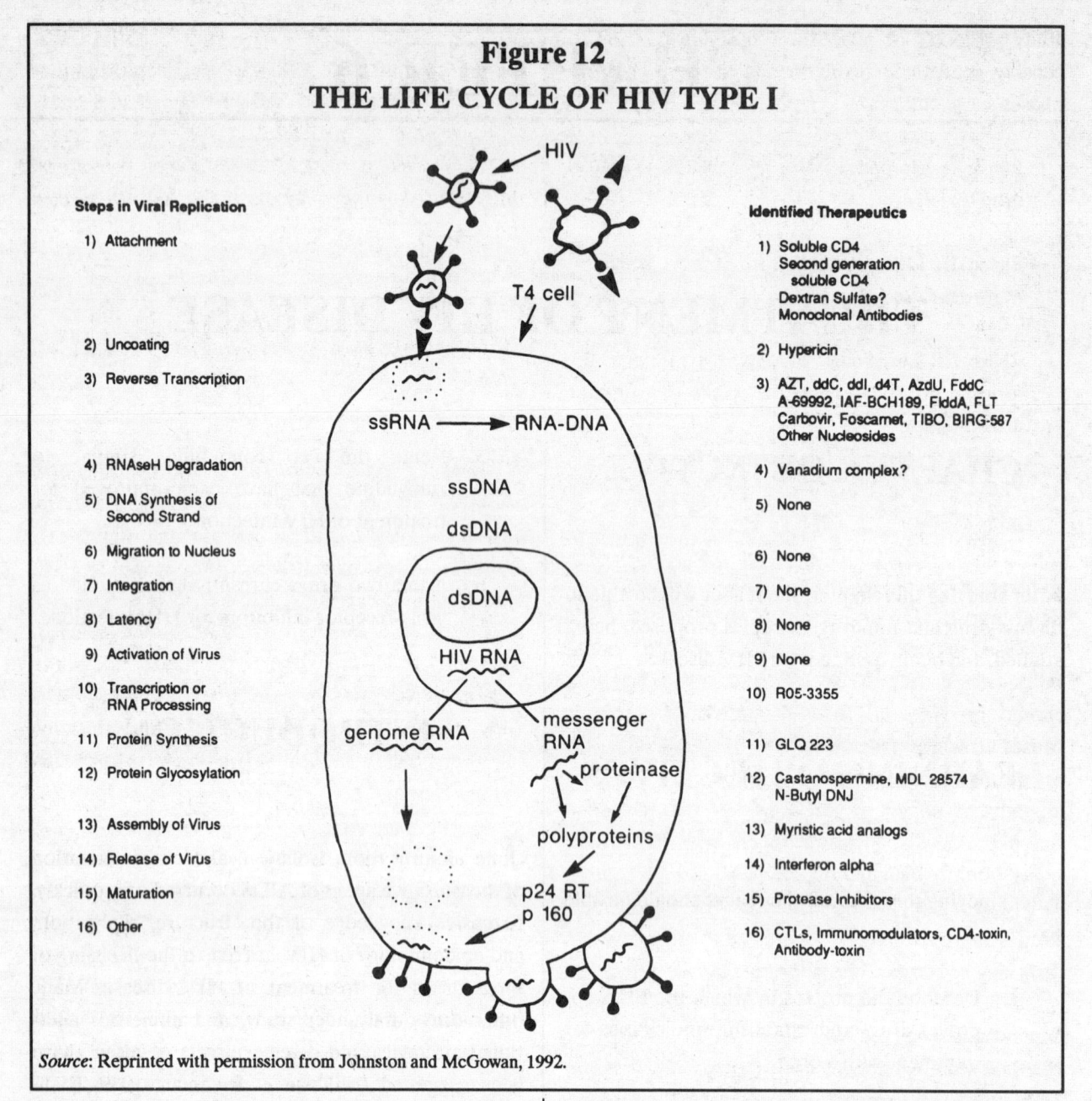

Steps in Viral Replication
1) Attachment
2) Uncoating
3) Reverse Transcription
4) RNAseH Degradation
5) DNA Synthesis of Second Strand
6) Migration to Nucleus
7) Integration
8) Latency
9) Activation of Virus
10) Transcription or RNA Processing
11) Protein Synthesis
12) Protein Glycosylation
13) Assembly of Virus
14) Release of Virus
15) Maturation
16) Other

Identified Therapeutics
1) Soluble CD4
   Second generation soluble CD4
   Dextran Sulfate?
   Monoclonal Antibodies
2) Hypericin
3) AZT, ddC, ddI, d4T, AzdU, FddC
   A-69992, IAF-BCH189, FIddA, FLT
   Carbovir, Foscarnet, TIBO, BIRG-587
   Other Nucleosides
4) Vanadium complex?
5) None
6) None
7) None
8) None
9) None
10) R05-3355
11) GLQ 223
12) Castanospermine, MDL 28574
    N-Butyl DNJ
13) Myristic acid analogs
14) Interferon alpha
15) Protease Inhibitors
16) CTLs, Immunomodulators, CD4-toxin, Antibody-toxin

Source: Reprinted with permission from Johnston and McGowan, 1992.

sible for long-term therapy, and (3) be safe and effective (Mildvan & Richman, 1989).

CLINICAL TRIALS

Numerous drugs have been proposed for treatment of HIV infection. Many of them were tested in earlier drug studies and found to be ineffective for the treatment of cancer or other life-threatening illnesses. It is not uncommon for a drug to be ineffective for one disease and effective for another.

Any drug used to treat any clinical problem, no matter what the problem is, must be approved by the FDA. Before a drug can be licensed for distribution to the general public, it must be tested. For clinical trials, pharmaceutical manufacturers, NIH, and the FDA collaborate in a well-documented four-phase process. Poor documentation or questions about

CHAPTER 6 —
TREATMENT OF HIV DISEASE

study protocols or procedures may prolong the licensing process or result in disapproval. The four phases are as follows:

Phase I: Limited studies in humans to detect drug toxicity

Phase II: Limited studies in humans to determine drug dosage

Phase III: Large-scale studies in humans to determine drug dosage and to begin determining drug efficacy

Phase IV: Further studies in humans to determine efficacy

FDA-approved drugs are continuously monitored to determine if (1) current use is appropriate, (2) a drug used to treat a broad range of conditions should be restricted to more specific use, and (3) a drug should be removed from the market because it causes unanticipated side effects. Physicians and others are requested to report immediately to the FDA any adverse effects or reactions that have not been noted previously. Information on side effects that occur often is included on the product insert sheets as a warning to future users. The use for which a drug is approved may be changed or restricted, or the drug may be removed from the market altogether.

Several decisions by the FDA have helped shorten the time required to get a drug approved. In October 1988, the FDA agreed to allow anti-AIDS medications to reach the market sooner, essentially cutting the approval time for these drugs in half. In addition, regulations on drug treatment for HIV-related infections have been relaxed. For example, the FDA agreed to make an experimental drug, trimetrexate, available for patients with PCP ("FDA: Drug Approval," 1988). Another policy change has shifted the burden of proof of effectiveness from the drug manufacturer to the FDA. Thus, the FDA must prove that a drug in question is not effective. Finally, in the fall of 1989, the FDA agreed to permit "parallel tracking" of drugs for HIV disease. Parallel tracking permits some patients to take a drug that is in a phase III study when the patients do not live near a center that is involved in the study or when their lives are so threatened that they may die if they do not receive the drug.

PROGRESS AGAINST HIV

When HIV was found to be the causative organism of AIDS, efforts turned to developing a vaccine against the virus and to designing chemotherapeutic regimens to treat persons already infected with HIV. A number of compounds active against retroviruses have been developed, and many are being tested in clinical trials. However, only a few, most still in the experimental phase, are available for treating HIV. Only three, zidovudine (AZT), dideoxycitidine (ddC), and dideoxyinosine (ddI), have been approved by the FDA.

None of these three rids the body of HIV, but they do decrease the amount of virus circulating in the bloodstream, which may help prolong life (Bakermann, 1988). Many of the currently studied drugs inhibit reverse transcriptase or prevent HIV from attaching to receptors for the virus on various cells (LaMontagne & Myers, 1987). A major problem in most clinical trials is that the virus becomes resistant to the drug being evaluated.

Other drugs being developed are immunomodulators, agents that can enhance or inhibit the immune response. The ones used for treatment of HIV disease stimulate the depressed immune system.

Many agents available outside the United States have been smuggled into the country through a transportation system nicknamed the "gray market." One such drug, widely used in Japan, is dextran sulfate. This cholesterol-lowering product showed promise in Japanese trials and is now sold without prescription (over the counter) in Japan (Hammer, 1988). Dextran sulfate has not been approved by the FDA. It is now in phase I and II clinical trials.

Project Inform, founded by Richard Delaney of San Francisco, is a source of information about experimental and gray-market drugs. The project publishes a newsletter about drugs that are being studied and drugs that may be therapeutic but for which no documented research is available. The goal of the project is to provide information about HIV infection and treatment to those infected and to the general public. The project does not determine the accuracy of the information, indicate whether it is proved by research, or screen for bias.

Drug studies require cooperation between the institution that enrolls and treats the patients (e.g., hospital, university), the company that makes the drug, the NIH, and the FDA. To facilitate the study of drugs for treatment of HIV disease and provide for consistency in the studies, the National Institute of Allergy and Infectious Diseases (NIAID) of the NIH established and funded coordinated programs in more than 100 cities. These programs are referred to as AIDS clinical trials units (ACTUs) or AIDS treatment and evaluation units (ATEUs). In some states, additional coordinated programs have been established and funded to study drugs and therapies not being evaluated in the ACTUs. One program in California is the California Collaborative Treatment Group (CCTG). Such groups may also exist in other states.

VIRUS-RECEPTOR INHIBITORS

The protein complex known as CD4 is the receptor for HIV. Interfering with the attachment of HIV to CD4 on the cell surface may be one way to prevent or treat HIV infection. Several treatments that interfere with attachment are currently being studied.

Monoclonal Antibodies

Monoclonal antibodies specific for (1) the virus or (2) receptors for the virus may prevent HIV from attaching to and infecting cells that have CD4 on their surface. In vitro studies are now being done to determine if this a possible method of treating HIV infection (Mildvan & Richman, 1989).

Neutralizing Antibodies

Infection with HIV leads to the production of antibodies against the virus. Normally, these antibodies are weak and ineffective in clearing or neutralizing the virus. Presumptive neutralization of HIV in passively immunized, symptomatic patients with HIV disease has been reported (Mildvan & Richman, 1989). These patients were given plasma from asymptomatic HIV-seropositive donors that had high levels of neutralizing antibody to HIV. The treatment appeared to suppress the virus, improve overall clinical status, and be well tolerated. Because of these promising results, passive immunotherapy is now being evaluated in several centers.

Recombinant Soluble CD4

Recombinant soluble CD4 is a genetically engineered polypeptide. It contains the portion of the CD4 molecule to which HIV attaches. In vitro, it inhibits HIV infection of CD4 cells by blocking attachment of HIV to CD4 on the cells' surface. In animal models, recombinant soluble CD4 appears to suppress the growth of HIV and improve bone marrow function. Intravenous treatment with this polypeptide is being studied at several ACTUs across the United States, and phase I trials for infants and children are being developed (Gomatos, Stamatos, & Schooley, 1992; Mildvan & Richman, 1989).

TAT Inhibitors

TAT is a protein that regulates replication of HIV. It is a transactivator. It stimulates the transcription of genes and affects their subsequent translation. Drugs that inhibit TAT can prevent replication of HIV. TAT is a good target for early drug intervention because the amount of drug needed to inhibit this protein may be less than the amount needed to inhibit the virus (Johnston & McGowan, 1992).

Immunotoxins

Immunotoxins consist of antibodies, hormones, or growth factors coupled to bacterial toxins or subunits of toxins. Immunotoxins that include ricin and *Pseudomonas* exotoxin have been used to treat HIV infection. Treatment has been beneficial in some patients and not in others (Gomatos et al., 1992).

Immunoadhesins

Immunoadhesins for treatment of HIV disease are designed to combine the binding specificity of CD4 with the effector domain of an immunoglobulin. One immunoadhesin (rsCD4IgG1) is in phase I clinical trials. The compound is being used to treat patients who have AIDS or severely symptomatic HIV infection (Gomatos et al., 1992).

Peptide T

Peptide T is an polypeptide. Its composition is similar to the composition of a glycoprotein found in the HIV envelope. Peptide T is thought to block binding of HIV to CD4 on the cell surface. In vitro, the peptide blocks infectivity of HIV. It is currently undergoing phase I and phase II studies (AIDS Clinical Trials, National Institutes of Health, Washington, DC, personal communication, June 1993; Mildvan & Richman, 1989).

AL-721

AL-721 is an antiviral agent with an unusual egg yolk and lecithin formula. First developed in Israel, it is now produced by Ethigen Corporation. In one study, AL-721 reduced the cholesterol content of some cell membranes. Changes in the cell membranes of CD4 cells lead to changes in the envelope membranes of HIV. Such changes may interfere with the attachment, penetration, and release of HIV (Grieco, Lange, Buimouici-Klein, & Reddy, 1988). In phase I studies, AL-721 was well tolerated over a broad range of doses but did not have any immunologic or antiviral effects. Some patients with HIV disease are now buying an over-the-counter form of the drug called "Eggs-Act." This substitute does not have the same formula as AL-721 (Mildvan & Richman, 1989).

Dextran Sulfate

Dextran sulfate seems to block the binding of HIV to CD4 and inhibit reverse transcriptase. It is not cytotoxic. In initial phase I studies, the oral form of the drug was poorly absorbed and had poor bioavailability. It also did not suppress the amount of viral antigens in the bloodstream to any great extent. Because dextran sulfate is a potent anticoagulant when administered intravenously, its use and effectiveness may be limited (Mildvan & Richman, 1989).

INHIBITORS OF REVERSE TRANSCRIPTASE

Once HIV has attached to and entered a cell, the cell uses HIV reverse transcriptase to make a DNA copy of viral RNA. Compounds that interfere with reverse transcriptase may prevent replication of the virus. An ideal inhibitor would reach high concentrations in CD4 cells, undergo metabolism, and inhibit reverse transcriptase without damaging the host cells' DNA (Mildvan & Richman, 1989).

Zidovudine

The first drug approved and available for HIV treatment was azidothymidine or zidovudine (Retrovir), better known as AZT. Zidovudine inhibits the replication and the cytopathic effects of HIV by inhibiting reverse transcriptase or by terminating elongation of viral DNA chains (Richman, 1988b). Treatment with zidovudine has been beneficial in patients with advanced HIV disease (Fischl, Richman, Grieco, & Gottlieb, 1987b; Sande & Volberding, 1992; Vella, Guilian, Pezzotti et al., 1992).

It is not uncommon for the CD4 count to increase during the first month of treatment (Vella et al., 1992). Prolonged use of zidovudine may result in HIV resistance to the drug (Fischl et al., 1987b). The current recommended dosage is 100 mg every 4 hr while awake.

Studies are being done to evaluate the effectiveness of even lower doses and to determine if viral resistance to the drug develops when lower doses are used. In addition, combination therapies in which zidovudine is used with another antiretroviral drug (such as acyclovir, alpha-interferon, ddI, and d4T) are being studied for their effectiveness against the virus and their role in preventing drug resistance.

Finally, initial studies in women, children, minority groups, and IDUs showed that treatment with zidovudine did not change the course of HIV infection. Continuing studies with larger groups of these subjects have shown that it does delay the progression of HIV disease (Howe, 1991d).

Treatment with zidovudine has significant side effects, and studies of its use in asymptomatic HIV-infected persons have not been completed. Therefore, treatment is limited to those with depressed immune systems. Currently, it is prescribed for patients whose CD4 count is less than 500 cells/mm^3 or in whom AIDS has been diagnosed.

Initial side effects are nausea, increased fatigue, headaches, flulike signs and symptoms, and generalized muscle and joint pains. These usually resolve after 4–8 weeks of treatment. The major side effect is bone marrow suppression. Patients should have CBCs and liver function tests done to determine if their bone marrow and liver are being affected. Zidovudine can cause leukopenia, neutropenia, anemia, and elevated levels of liver enzymes. For this reason, patients should not be started on AZT if their neutrophil count is less than 1,000, their hemoglobin level is less than 9.0 g/dL, or their levels of liver enzymes are five times greater than normal (Richman et al., 1987). The effects of long-term treatment with zidovudine are still under investigation, but studies indicate that lower doses cause fewer long-term side effects. One long-term side effect is viral resistance to the drug. If this happens, additional medication should be included in the treatment regimen.

Dideoxyinosine (ddI)

Dideoxyinosine (Didanosine, Videx) is another compound similar to zidovudine and ddC. It was approved by the FDA in October 1991. Information about this drug before its approval raised hopes among patients with HIV disease. For those who could no longer tolerate zidovudine, ddI offered a treatment regimen free of hematologic and gastrointestinal side effects. Studies of ddI are still in progress, but many of the early hopes have been dashed because it has neurologic and pancreatic side effects (Mildvan & Richman, 1989). It is used to treat adults with advanced HIV disease who have been treated with zidovudine (Bartlett, 1992).

Didanosine comes in chewable tablets or a buffered powder for oral solution and must be taken on an empty stomach. The tablets can be crushed and dissolved in an ounce of water to decrease the dryness in the mouth caused by chewing the tablets. The dosages below are based on body weight.

The most serious side effects of ddI are pancreatitis and peripheral neuropathy. Patients taking ddI should have their serum levels of amylase and lipase monitored. However, increases may not be evident until after an episode of pancreatitis occurs. If progressive increases in the amylase level occur, use of ddI should be stopped, and the patient should be monitored closely. Use of the drug should also be stopped if abdominal pain develops or the patient has nausea or vomiting (Fischl, 1992).

Additional side effects include dry mouth and diarrhea. The diarrhea is caused by the antacid used to buffer the ddI. It usually occurs when treatment is started. If it persists, antidiarrheal agents may be necessary.

Dideoxycytidine (ddC)

Dideoxycytidine (Zalcitabine, Hivid) is similar to zidovudine. It can be taken orally. It also is an inhibitor of reverse transcriptase. In initial studies in humans, it reduced the amount of viral antigens in the bloodstream. The drug was approved by the FDA in June 1992. It is used only in combination with zidovudine in patients with advanced HIV disease who have signs of clinical deterioration. Caution should be used when treatment with ddC is started, especially if the patient complains of pain, numbness, or tingling in the lower extremities. Patients with evidence of peripheral neuropathy should not use ddC.

The current recommended dosage of ddC is 0.75 mg orally every 8 hr along with 200 mg of zidovudine. The most significant side effect is dose-related peripheral neuropathy (Bartlett, 1992). Studies are now under way to determine if use of zidovudine and ddC in alternating combinations will increase the effectiveness of the drugs and reduce toxic side effects and the development of drug resistance (Richman, 1988b).

d4T

The compound d4T is another dideoxynucleoside (thymidine) analogue. It inhibits HIV replication by inducing premature termination of viral DNA chains. The analogue was made available in October 1992 through the FDA's parallel tracking policy. It is used to treat patients who have not responded to or are intolerant of zidovudine or ddI. Major side ef-

Patient's Weight (kg)	Chewable Tablets (mg, twice a day)	Buffered Powder (mg, twice a day)
>75	300	375
50–74	200	250
35–49	125	167

fects include peripheral neuropathy, increased levels of liver enzymes, headaches, and nausea (American Foundation for AIDS Research [AmFAR], Spring 1992a).

Suramin

Suramin is the hexasodium salt derivative of naphthalene trisulfonic acid. It was first produced in 1916 by the Bayer Company as an antiparasitic drug. It is still widely used in Africa to treat trypanosomiasis and onchocerciasis. Suramin affects a wide variety of enzymes in many organisms. It inhibits HIV reverse transcriptase, which reduces replication. It may also interfere with viral binding to CD4-positive cells (Mildvan & Richman, 1989; Wormser et al., 1987).

Suramin has a number of unpleasant side effects. It can cause rash, fever, proteinuria, elevated levels of liver transaminase, pyuria, and a burning sensation in the arms and legs. In one study, 33% of patients had adrenal insufficiency after using this drug (Wormser et al., 1987). To date, toxic effects have exceeded benefits for the dose and schedule used (Richman, 1988a).

Trisodium Phosphonoformate

Trisodium phosphonoformate (PFA, Foscarnet, Foscavir) is an antiviral agent that was first synthesized in 1924. The topical form has been used in Sweden since 1980 to treat mucocutaneous HSV infections (Wormser et al., 1987). The drug inhibits viral DNA polymerases of all human herpesviruses, including HSV, CMV, and EBV. It also inhibits the RNA polymerase of influenza virus. In clinical trials, CMV infections have been more susceptible than HIV infections to this agent.

The major drawbacks of trisodium phosphonoformate are its short serum half-life, poor concentration in cells, and poor absorption of oral doses. As a result, continuous large-volume intravenous infusion is necessary to obtain adequate plasma levels. Major side effects include phlebitis at the infusion site, reversible renal impairment, anemia, hypocalcemia, and hypophosphatemia (Mildvan & Richman, 1989; Sande & Volberding, 1992).

Ampligen

Ampligen, or mismatched RNA (manufactured by DuPont), was thought to be a promising anti-HIV agent. In trials in humans, adverse side effects were limited to flulike signs and symptoms. However, in phase II clinical trials, the drug did not have any effect on the progression to AIDS (Carter, Strayer, Brodsky, & Lewin, 1987; Cohen, Sande, & Volberding, 1990). Additional studies are under way.

OTHER ANTIVIRAL AGENTS

Currently, more than 60 antiviral or immunomodulating agents are being tested by drug companies, the NIH, and investigators across the country. Thus far, none has come close to approval.

Ribavirin

Ribavirin (Virazole), made by Viratek/ICN Pharmaceuticals, is a synthetic nucleoside derivative of the antibiotic pyrazomycin. It has a broad spectrum of activity against both DNA and RNA viruses in vitro (Wormser et al., 1987). After it is phosphorylated intracellularly, this compound interferes with an essential step of viral messenger RNA. It is thought to resemble guanosine (Vogt, Hartshorn, Furman, & Chou, 1987). The results of studies with ribavirin have been contradictory. Investigations to determine its effectiveness are still in progress (Richman, 1988a). Anemia has been the only important side effect noted.

Ribavirin is not licensed in the United States for treatment of HIV disease, but some patients have traveled to Mexico to buy it, where it is freely available. Aerosolized ribavirin is effective for treatment of respiratory syncytial virus infections. This dosage form is licensed for this purpose in the United States.

Interferon

It is unclear how alpha-interferon inhibits HIV replication. It may slow down the release of mature, infectious virus (Cohen et al., 1990). Alpha-interferon must be given parenterally, and it does not readily cross the blood-brain barrier. Specific side effects include fever, malaise, myalgias, and bone marrow suppression.

In a recent study in Kenya, HIV-positive patients treated with oral doses of alpha-interferon (known as Kemron) had increases in the number of CD4 cells. To date, no other study has shown similar increases in CD4 counts.

Compound Q

Compound Q is a product of a cucumber root plant found in China. In vitro, it kills HIV-infected macrophages and blocks replication of HIV in CD4 cells (Sande & Volberding, 1992). Serious side effects include flulike signs and symptoms, myalgias, and toxic effects in the central nervous system potentially leading to stupor or coma or both.

IMMUNOTHERAPY

A selective abnormality develops in CD4 helper-inducer T lymphocytes when these cells are infected with HIV (Bakermann, 1988). Immunotherapy is designed to help rebuild or enhance the damaged immune system.

Inosine Pranobex

Inosine pranobex (Isoprinosine), produced by Newport Pharmaceuticals, is indicated for asymptomatic HIV disease, progressive lymphadenopathy, and HIV infection. In vitro, inosine pranobex enhances lymphocyte proliferation, macrophage activation, and other immune functions. Studies on this drug are under way in the United States, Australia, and Scandinavia. To date, none of the results have indicated that it is effective in persons with HIV disease.

COMBINATION THERAPY

Treatment of HIV infection with a combination of drugs is a logical strategy to explore. Many of the anti-HIV agents act at different steps in replication, so a combination of agents may lead to enhanced efficacy and fewer toxic effects. Combination therapy may also help reduce drug resistance.

Some of the drugs currently being used in combination therapy are zidovudine and acyclovir, zidovudine and ddC, and zidovudine and recombinant soluble CD4. Future combinations could include alpha-interferon, alpha-interferon, trisodium phosphonoformate, and dextran sulfate.

Studies are in progress to evaluate the safety and immunologic and antiviral effects of combination therapy with zidovudine and ddC or ddI. A recent study showed that zidovudine and ddC given simultaneously caused no unexpected side effects and appeared to be well tolerated (Meng et al., 1991). The greatest increase in CD4 counts occurred at dosages of 600 mg/day of zidovudine and 0.005 or 0.01 mg/kg per day of ddC. Development of drug resistance was not determined.

Some physicians think that patients taking zidovudine who have rapidly declining CD4 counts should be switched to ddI or take a combination of zidovudine and ddC. In patients who have been taking zidovudine for more than 18 months and who have a decreasing CD4 count, switching to ddI appears to increase the number of CD4 cells and the patient's overall well-being. This is especially true when the number of CD4 cells is rapidly decreasing.

Now that ddI and ddC have been approved by the FDA, more use of combination or alternating drug therapy is likely. Another combination therapy being studied is zidovudine and alpha-interferon. Preliminary results have indicated that this combination is effective in sustaining CD4 counts. Some evidence suggests that this combination is active against Kaposi's sarcoma ("The Advent of," 1991).

VACCINES

Vaccines are designed to produce an initial immune response to an antigen and establish antigen-specific "memory cells." When the antigen or a pathogen bearing the antigen enters the body a second time, whether 1 month or 1 year later, the memory cells are activated, and a secondary immune response occurs. The secondary response leads to destruction or inhibition of the antigen or pathogen, thus preventing infection or disease.

Once the cause of AIDS was identified, the race to develop a vaccine began. In a well-publicized experiment, Daniel Zagury, a French immunologist, injected himself with an experimental vaccine that he later tested in a series of healthy volunteers. He reported that an immune state against HIV can be obtained in humans (Leonard, Zagury, Desportes, & Bernard, 1988).

Current approaches to the development of HIV vaccines are based on previous experience with viral vaccines (polio and measles) and on new information gained in molecular biology and immunology. Unfortunately, even though a great deal of information about HIV was gathered in a short time, little is known about how the virus replicates or about the immune responses to HIV infection in humans.

The rationale for developing a vaccine is that use of the vaccine would induce an immune response that would confer resistance to HIV or the ability to recover from infection with HIV. The response could have humoral or cellular components or both. The vaccines that have been tested so far have produced both humoral and cellular responses. However, none has caused any change in the natural history of the virus (Hendry & Quinnan, 1989).

Development of an HIV vaccine continues to be a high research priority because of the high prevalence of HIV disease throughout the world. However, several obstacles must be dealt with. These include (1) the lack of knowledge about what constitutes protective immunity against HIV, (2) lack of knowledge about the way HIV integrates into the cellular genome, and (3) various ethical issues of conducting phase II and phase III clinical trials. Despite these difficulties, significant advances have been made, and numerous vaccine trials are currently being conducted.

More than 30 different possible vaccines are now being tested. Any one of them could be available for use by the turn of the century. A trial with a vaccine called HGP-30, which is purely synthetic and contains no live virus or genetic material, will be done in Britain. HGP-30 was developed in the United States by Viral Technologies, but Britain granted approval for its use before the FDA did ("Are Investigational Drugs," 1988). The Salk Institute is also working on a vaccine to be used in persons with HIV infection. This vaccine is said to increase circulating antibodies

CHAPTER 6 —
TREATMENT OF HIV DISEASE

against HIV. The antibodies combine with HIV and make the virus inactive.

Another human trial has been approved for an experimental vaccine developed by Bristol-Myers Company. The agent in this vaccine is vaccinia virus, which is used to immunize against smallpox. It has been genetically engineered to bear antigens from the outer coat of HIV (Bakermann, 1988).

OTHER THERAPIES

Two patients with HIV disease had their blood heated to 110°F outside the body and then reinfused in an effort to kill the virus. In the patients involved, Kaposi's sarcoma was the only AIDS-related disorder. The physician who performed the procedure claims that the number of white blood cells steadily increased and that the sarcomas shrank after the treatment. The efficacy and safety of the procedure are unproved. However, an NIAID team found that the treatment offered no clinical, immunologic, or virologic benefits to the two patients ("Clinical Use of Hyperthermia," 1990).

WHERE TO GET TREATMENT

Numerous ACTUs can be found throughout the United States (Figure 13). In addition, many re-

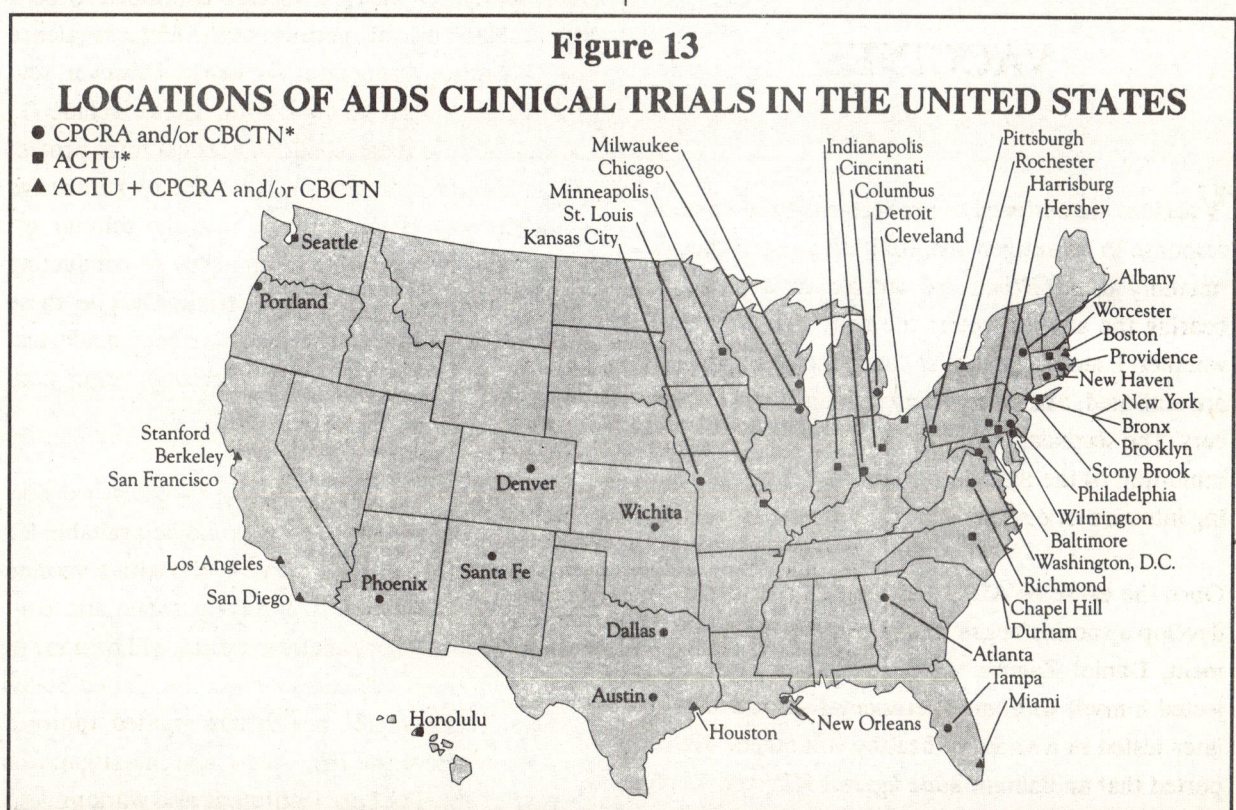

Figure 13
LOCATIONS OF AIDS CLINICAL TRIALS IN THE UNITED STATES

- ● CPCRA and/or CBCTN*
- ■ ACTU*
- ▲ ACTU + CPCRA and/or CBCTN

The following sites were also included in clinical trials: ACTU: Chicago, IL; Denver, CO; New Brunswick, NJ; New Orleans, LA; Washington, DC. CBCTN: Redwood City, CA; Sherman Oaks, CA. ACTU/CPCRA/CBCTN: Newark, NJ.

Source: Portions of the publication, "AIDS Clinical Care" are reprinted by permission. ACC (c) 3:24, 3:32. Massachusetts Medical Society. All rights reserved.

search grants have been awarded to various outpatient clinics, medical centers, and universities.

Patients with HIV infection who are interested in participating in these programs should contact their nearest university or AIDS project to find out where the ACTUs and other research centers are located. Each research project has specific criteria for participation, and all potential subjects are screened for suitability.

Chapter 7 discusses treatment of the opportunistic infections, tumors, and dementia associated with HIV disease.

EXAM QUESTIONS

Chapter 6

Questions 44 -47

44. Which of the following is a drug approved by the Food and Drug Administration for treatment of HIV infection?

    a. **Zidovudine** ✓
    b. Acyclovir
    c. Ribavirin
    d. Alpha-interferon

45. What two new inhibitors of reverse transcriptase are being used to treat HIV infection?

    a. Dideoxyinosine (ddI) and ribavirin
    b. Ribavirin and acyclovir
    c. Acyclovir and dideoxycytidine (ddC)
    d. **Dideoxycytidine and dideoxyinosine** ✓

46. Soluble CD4 belongs to which category of experimental drugs for treatment of HIV infection?

    a. **Reverse transcriptase inhibitors** ✓
    b. Virus-receptor inhibitors
    c. Monoclonal antibodies
    d. Vaccines

47. What are three side effects of zidovudine therapy?

    a. Rash, nausea, and increased white blood cell count
    b. **Generalized muscle pain, joint pain, and leukopenia** ✓
    c. Hemoglobin more than 11 g/dl, decreased kidney function, and thrombocytopenia
    d. Photophobia, muscle pain, and decreased CD4 count

CHAPTER 7

MEDICAL MANAGEMENT OF OPPORTUNISTIC INFECTIONS, TUMORS, AND AIDS DEMENTIA COMPLEX

CHAPTER OBJECTIVE

After studying this chapter, the reader will be able to discuss the opportunistic infections, tumors, and dementia associated with HIV disease and current medical treatments of these disorders.

LEARNING OBJECTIVES

After studying this chapter, the reader should be able to

1. Define the term opportunistic infection.

2. Name the second most common protozoal infection in persons with HIV disease.

3. Indicate the signs and symptoms of *Pneumocystis carinii* pneumonia.

4. Specify the treatment of choice for pneumocystis pneumonia.

5. Differentiate between *Mycobacterium avium-intracellulare* and *Mycobacterium tuberculosis*.

6. Name three drugs used to treat infection caused by *M. avium-intracellulare*.

7. Indicate the medications most often used to treat cryptococcal infections.

8. Describe how an organ responds to infection with *Toxoplasma*.

9. Describe the most common side effects of the drugs used to treat toxoplasmosis.

10. Specify which organisms most often cause diarrhea in persons with HIV disease.

11. Name the most common opportunistic viral infection in persons with HIV disease.

12. Indicate the most common site of the most common viral opportunistic infection in persons with HIV disease.

13. Specify the organ or organ systems that cytomegalovirus (CMV) affects.

14. Name the drug that is licensed for treatment of CMV infections and describe its side effects.

15. Name the microorganism that causes shingles.

16. Indicate the side effects of the drug acyclovir (Zovirax).

17. Indicate the tumors most commonly seen in persons with HIV disease.

18. Indicate which group of persons most often had Kaposi's sarcoma before HIV disease became widespread.

19. Specify the four types of lymphoma seen in persons with HIV disease.

20. Describe the signs and symptoms of the early and late stages of AIDS dementia complex (ADC).

21. Describe the current treatment of ADC.

ASSESSMENT OF PERSONS WITH HIV DISEASE

As more effective methods of preventing and treating disorders associated with HIV disease are developed, the quality of life of those infected with HIV will improve. Many health care providers recommend assessment of everyone who is seropositive for HIV. The purpose is to determine the extent of the associated immunodeficiency and to detect opportunistic infections, tumors, or other disorders. Assessments should be done on the initial visit and then every 6–12 months.

Initial assessment usually takes place in the ambulatory care setting, but it may not be done until the patient has been hospitalized for treatment of an acute condition. In either case, certain information should be obtained, and certain laboratory tests should be done. For patients early in the course of HIV disease, the results provide baseline information on immune status and previous or current infections.

Initial screening laboratory tests should include the following: CBC, including differential and number of platelets; chemistry panel that includes renal, liver, and pancreatic function tests; CD4 count; RPR or VDRL tests; determination of serum levels of hepatitis B antigen and antibodies to HBV; and tests for toxoplasmosis if the CD4 count is less than 200 cells/mm^3 or if toxoplasmic encephalitis is a potential diagnosis. An initial chest radiograph is helpful but not crucial. A skin test for mycobacteria (PPD) should also be done. Skin tests for *Histoplasma* and cryptococci should be done if the person has lived in an area where these two organisms exist. Skin tests with tetanus toxoid and with antigens for *Candida* and mumps will help determine if the person is anergic.

After the initial evaluation, HIV-infected persons should be placed on an ongoing program of prophylaxis that begins with pneumococcal pneumonia vaccine and routine influenza vaccine. Patients with a PPD reaction of 5 mm or greater should start a 12-month course of treatment with isoniazid (300 mg/day). Homosexual men who are sexually active, IDUs who are still using drugs (other than drugs for treatment of disease), and sexual partners of HBV carriers should receive hepatitis B vaccine (Bartlett, 1992).

Patients with HIV infection who are asymptomatic should be seen at least every 6 months. Assessment should include CBC, including differential; CD4 count; chemistry panel; history; and physical examination. This monitoring helps detect subtle changes that can occur over time.

Currently, treatment of HIV infection is confined to three antiretroviral drugs: zidovudine, ddI, and ddC. The CD4 count is the laboratory indicator most frequently used to determine when antiretroviral therapy should be started. The patient's clinical picture should also be considered. Table 11 provides a synopsis of staging and treatment of HIV infection.

Generally, when the CD4 count is less than 500 cells/mm^3 on two consecutive occasions, zidovudine should be started (as long as blood parameters are within recommended limits). PCP prophylaxis with Septra DS (sulfamethoxazole/trimethoprim), dapsone, or pentamidine should be started when the CD4 count is 200 cells/mm^3 or the number of CD4 cells is less than 20% of the total number of lymphocytes. If the patient has had a splenectomy, PCP prophylaxis should be started when the CD4 count reaches 300 cells/mm^3 or 20% of the total number of lymphocytes.

Health care providers are also recommending that prophylaxis against toxoplasmosis should be started when the patient has antibodies to *Toxoplasma* antibodies, and the CD4 count is less than 200 cells/mm^3. Pyrimethamine (Daraprim) alone or with sulfadoxine (Fansidar) ("Primary Prophylaxis," 1991; Remington & Araujo, 1992), sulfadiazine, or clindamycin (Cleocin) is used for secondary prophylaxis and may be helpful in providing primary prophylaxis. Some evidence indicates that Septra given for PCP prophylaxis may also prevent toxoplasmosis.

Drugs that provide effective treatment of primary coccidioidomycosis and histoplasmosis and secondary prophylaxis are being evaluated. For coccidioidomycosis, the most common ones are amphotericin B for primary treatment and fluconazole (Diflucan), ketoconazole (Nizoral), and reduced dosages of amphotericin B for secondary prophylaxis (Girard, Pocidolo, & Murray, 1991). Amphotericin B is recommended for primary and secondary treatment of histoplasmosis. An alternative for secondary treatment is ketoconazole. Itraconazole (Sporanox) was approved in October 1992 by the FDA for treatment of histoplasmosis and blastomycosis. It is thought to be more effective than ketoconazole in these two infections. It is also being used to treat aspergillosis and eosinophilia folliculitis (Howe, 1992b).

OPPORTUNISTIC INFECTIONS

The primary cause of morbidity and mortality in patients infected with HIV is opportunistic infections. These infections occur because the immune system is weakened or destroyed.

"Opportunistic" is an excellent term for the infections that afflict persons who have HIV disease. The organisms that cause these infections exist in the everyday environment. They are not usually pathogens. In a person with a normal, healthy immune system, they do not ordinarily cause disease. However, once

Table 11
Staging and Treatment of HIV Infection

Disease Stage	CD4 Count (cells/mm^3)	Treatment
Early	>500	Currently, no treatment indicated. Monitor CD4 count every 3–6 months. Update immunizations.
Middle	200–500	Prescribe zidovudine, 500 mg/day in divided doses. Monitor CBC every 2 weeks for 1 month, then once a month for 2 months, then every 2 months if patient stable. Monitor CD4 counts every 3 months. Do not start zidovudine therapy in an asymptomatic person without documentation of positive antibody tests. Do not start zidovudine therapy at patient's first visit.
Later	<200	Prescribe zidovudine, 500 mg/day (e.g., patients with AIDS dementia complex). Monitor same as in middle stage disease. Obtain other laboratory tests as indicated by patient's clinical condition. Start prophylaxis for *Pneumocystis carinii* pneumonia: Trimethoprim/sulfamethoxazole, one double-strength tablet daily, or dapsone, 50–100 mg daily, or inhaled pentamidine, 300 mg monthly

Source: Adapted from Clement & Hollander, 1992.

the immune system is compromised or weakened, they can cause infection.

Persons with HIV disease are not the only ones who have opportunistic infections. The infections can develop in anyone whose immune system is compromised or suppressed. This includes those who have had radiation or chemotherapy, those who have had treatment to prevent the rejection of a transplanted organ, and those who have genetically acquired immunodeficiency. Often these infections are more severe and persistent in persons with HIV disease than in other immunocompromised patients. Recurrences are frequent, despite repeated treatment (Pratt, 1986).

Opportunistic infections in persons with HIV disease are different from those in patients with other types of immunodeficiency. The clinical signs and symptoms are blunted and more insidious (DeVita, Hellman, & Rosenberg, 1985). The impairment in CD4 cells caused by HIV leads to abnormalities in both humoral and cellular immune responses, including failure to produce granulomas and unreliable serologic responses (Selwyn, 1986b). For example, *Pneumocystis* infections may develop quietly over weeks or months in persons with HIV infection. In transplant patients, the same infection would progress over a few days. In persons with HIV disease, CMV causes more disseminated disease and produces complications such as esophageal ulcers, malabsorption colitis, and adrenal insufficiency (Drew, Buhles, & Erlich, 1988). In addition, serologic tests for CMV and *Toxoplasma* become unreliable. Levels of antibody do not increase enough to be detected or increase no further during reactivation or no primary antibody response occurs (Selwyn, 1986a).

Approximately 80% of all patients with advanced HIV disease will have an episode of pneumocystis pneumonia. In adults without HIV infection, the rate is 1% or less. *Mycobacterium avium-intracellulare* (MAI) infection is also rare in persons without HIV infection. Fewer than 20 cases of disseminated MAI infection were reported in the literature before 1979 (Kovacs & Masur, 1988). Other illnesses that were rarely seen before the HIV epidemic have also become more common.

Researchers have been trying to develop drugs that would prevent or eliminate opportunistic infections. Successful treatment would reduce the number of deaths and improve the length and quality of life of all patients whose immune systems are weakened or suppressed. However, funds for studies of drug treatment of opportunistic infections have not been a priority. So far, most research funds have been used to find drugs to treat HIV infection or to develop a vaccine for HIV. As the epidemic has progressed, health care providers have become more outspoken about the need for studies that seek new treatments for opportunistic infections.

HIV disease is a protracted illness that usually involves several opportunistic infections. At times, patients and health care providers alike may wish to ignore or deny evidence of a new or recurring opportunistic infection. However, it is imperative that each episode of infection be recognized and treated early. Although AIDS is not curable today, its signs and symptoms can be managed to lengthen and improve the patient's quality of life. AIDS is now viewed as a long-term illness with peaks and valleys similar to those seen in other chronic illnesses such as lung disease and hypertension (Kovacs & Masur, 1988).

The major infections found in persons infected with HIV are listed in Table 12 (p.90). Patients often have more than one opportunistic infection at a time. Others may have only one opportunistic infection during the entire course of their HIV disease. The reason one infection rather than another develops is unknown. Some opportunistic infections are a reflection of environmental exposure, which may differ according to the patient's geographic location, history, and life-style. Toxoplasmosis is an example of such an infection. Some scientists have speculated that

Table 12
THE INFECTIONS OF AIDS

Type	Causative Agent or Infection
Bacterial	*Mycobacterium avium-intracellulare*
	Mycobacterium tuberculosis
	Nocardia
	Salmonella
	Shigella flexnerii
	Legionella species
	Listeria monocytogenes
Fungal	*Candida albicans*
	Aspergillus (central nervous system)
	Cryptococcus neoformans
	Coccidioides immitis
	Histoplasma capsulatum
	Tineal infections
Protozoal	*Pneumocystis carinii*
	Strongyloides stercolaris
	Cryptosporidium species
	Toxoplasma gondii
	Giardia lamblia
	Entamoeba histolytica
	Isospora belli
Viral	Cytomegalovirus
	Herpes simplex virus
	Epstein-Barr virus
	Papovavirus

differences in the virus itself may account for the development of an opportunistic infection.

The opportunistic infections most frequently encountered in HIV disease are discussed in the following pages. Only the most common infections and their primary treatments are presented (see Table 13, p.91–92 for a summary). More detailed information can be found in the references listed in the Bibliography.

Protozoal Opportunistic Infections

Pneumocystis carinii

Pneumocystis carinii pneumonia (PCP) is the most common opportunistic infection seen in persons infected with HIV. The causative agent is thought to be a protozoan found in mammals. The organism is transmitted by the respiratory route. Most healthy children have acquired it by the time they are 4 years old (Flaskerud & Ungvarski, 1992). The infection is latent until sufficient immunodeficiency occurs. Then it becomes active.

The organism usually affects the lungs, although it has been found in the liver, spleen, and lymph nodes. When the protozoan is found in organs other than the lungs, the illness is called disseminated pneumocystosis.

Signs and Symptoms. Pneumocystis pneumonia frequently has a slow, subtle onset, with signs and symptoms occurring over weeks or months. With the advent of PCP prophylaxis, in some HIV-infected persons, full-blown PCP may not develop for several months. Signs and symptoms are fever, chills, sweats, dry cough, chest tightness, shortness of breath, and progressive fatigue.

Diagnostic Evaluation. Laboratory tests should include CBC, with differential and platelets; a chemistry panel, including renal and liver function tests and electrolytes; partial thromboplastin time (PTT) and prothrombin time (PT); arterial blood gas (ABG) analysis; and chest radiograph. (The PTT and PT are done in preparation for bronchoscopy.)

Induced sputums should be obtained in the early morning. If sputum tests are negative for PCP, then bronchoscopy should be done. Some practitioners advocate performing gallium scans before or along with bronchoscopy. However, increased pulmonary uptake of gallium can also indicate other lung infections and is not specific for PCP. Pulmonary function tests may also be done.

CHAPTER 7 — MEDICAL MANAGEMENT OF OPPORTUNISTIC INFECTIONS, TUMORS, AND AIDS DEMENTIA COMPLEX

Table 13
TREATMENT OF OPPORTUNISTIC INFECTIONS

Infection	Drug(s)	Dosage and duration	Comments
Pneumocysitis carinii pneumonia	Sulfamethoxazole/ trimethoprim or Pentamidine	100 mg/kg per day for 14–21 days 20 mg/kg per day 4 mg/kg daily intramuscularly or intravenously	Requires prophylaxis Sulfamethoxozole/ trimethoprim + 300 mg aerosolized by mouth four times a day
	Dapsone/Trimethoprim Clindamycin	100 mg; 20 mg/kg per day 750 mg four times a day or 900 mg three times a day	50 mg four times a day By mouth or intravenously
	Primaguine	30 mg (base) orally four times a day	Check levels of glucose-6-phosphate dehydrogenase Watch for methemoglobinemia
Cryptococcal meningitis	Amphotericin B and	0.4–0.6 mg/kg per day for 6 weeks 100 mg/kg per day	Requires prophylaxis
	Flucytosine or Fluconazole	100–500 mg/day orally	Contraindicated if low WBC count
Toxoplasmosis	Sulfadiazine sodium and Pyrimethamine Leucovorin* Clindamycin	4 g/day orally for 6 weeks 25–50 mg/day orally 5–10 mg/day orally 300–900 mg every 6–8 hours	Reduce doses to 2 g of sulfadiazine, 25 mg of pyrimethamine Continue indefinitely
Histoplasmosis	Amphotericin B	0.25–1.50 mg/kg per day intravenously	By central line for a total of 1.5–3.0 g
	Fluconazole Itraconazole	200–400 mg/day orally 200–400 mg/day orally	Prophylaxis dose Prophylaxis dose
Mycobacterium avium-intracellulare infection	Isoniazide (INH)* Rifampin* Ethambutol* Clofazamine* Ciprofloxacin* Azithromycin* Clarithromycin* Rifabutin* Amikacin	300 mg/day 600 mg/day 800–1200 mg/day 200 mg/day 1000–1500 mg/day 500–1000 mg orally twice a day 500–1000 mg orally twice a day 300–600 mg/day orally 7.5 mg/kg twice a day intravenously or intramuscularly or 10 mg/kg per day intravenously or intramuscularly	Usually two or more drugs are given at one time No documented evidence to suggest treatment is effective In prophylaxis studies Observe for ototoxic or nephrotoxic effects
Mycobacterium tuberculosis infection	Isoniazide (INH) Rifampin Ethambutol Pyrazinamide	300 mg/day 600 mg/day 800–1200 mg/day or 25 mg/kg per day 25 mg/kg per day in three to four divided doses	Use three of these four for the first 2 months, then use only INH and rifampin for 6–12 months Monitor for development of drug resistance
Cryptosporidiosis	Azithromycin* Clarithromycin* No clearly effective agent	Dosages not known	

*Indications for use unclear or unproved

Table 13 (Continued)

Infection	Drug(s)	Dosage and duration	Comments
Oral candidiasis	Clotrimazole troche (10 mg) or Nystatin swish Ketoconazole Fluconazole	One to five troches/day until resolved 500,000 U four times a day 200 mg once or twice a day for 5–10 days 100–500 mg/day	Based on amount of thrush Return to clotrimazole after treated
Esophageal candidiasis	Ketoconazole Fluconazole	200 mg twice a day for 10–14 days 100–500 mg/day	
Vaginal candidiasis	Clortrimazole (Gyne-Lotrimin) Ketoconazole Fluconazole	One tab or applicator at bedtime 400 mg/day for 14 days 200–400 mg/day	For 2 weeks If clortimazole fails. Give for 5 days each month for 6 months. If ketoconazole fails to control infection
Cytomegalovirus infection	Ganciclovir (DHPG) Foscarnet	5 mg/kg twice a day intravenously for 14 days 3-5 mg/kg per day intravenously 5 days each week 60 mg/kg three times a day for 2–3 weeks Then 90 mg/kg four times a day	Initial dose Maintenance may vary according to site of infection Requires monitoring of renal function and chemistries Requires central line and controlled infusion
Herpes simplex virus infection	Acyclovir Foscarnet	200 mg orally five times a day for 7–10 days 60 mg/kg three times a day for 2–3 weeks	Consider twice a day maintenance if frequent recurrence
Herpes zoster virus infection	Acyclovir*	10 mg/kg per day intravenously for 5–10 days	Indication or effectiveness not clear

*Indications for use unclear or unproved

If this is a patient's first opportunistic infection, the WBC will probably be normal or low, with increased numbers of neutrophils and bands. Normocytic anemia and an increase in the level of lactic dehydrogenase are common.

Serial chest radiographs show slowly progressive diffuse interstitial infiltrates in both lungs. Some practitioners consider the gradual loss of vertebral markings on lateral chest films diagnostic for PCP. As the pneumonia clears, the vertebral markings become more prominent again.

Analysis of ABGs may show a decrease in the PaO2 to less than 70 mm Hg. Often the ABG values are in the 60s and 50s. Anyone with a PaO2 less than 75 mm Hg and an arterial-alveolar (AA) gradient greater than 25 should be admitted to the hospital. Pulmonary function tests may be of some help in the diagnosis. PCP causes a decrease in diffusing capacity for carbon monoxide.

Definitive diagnosis is made by obtaining the protozoal cysts from sputum or on the basis of findings on bronchial lavage or biopsy.

Treatment. Initial treatment is oxygen therapy and trimethoprim (15–20 mg/kg per day) and sulfamethoxazole (75–100 mg/kg per day) [Bactrim, Septra, cotrimoxazole, TMP/SMX] given in three to four equally divided doses either intravenously or orally for 21 days.

Intravenous pentamidine may be used if the patient is allergic to or cannot tolerate Septra. The dosage is 4 mg/kg per day in a single dose for 14–21 days. Inhaled pentamidine has been used as the initial treatment, but there is no documented evidence of increased efficacy when this formulation is used.

Oral dapsone and trimethoprim may be used when patients cannot tolerate Septra or pentamidine or when PCP is mild and outpatient therapy is desired. The dosages are 100 mg of dapsone and 15 mg/kg trimethoprim once a day. This treatment is not recommended for those with glucose-6-phosphatase dehydrogenase (G6PD) deficiency, and screening for G6PD deficiency should be done before treatment with dapsone is started.

Another alternative therapy for PCP is a regimen of oral clindamycin (Cleocin) and primaquine. Treatment response rates for these two drugs are similar to the rate for treatment with TMP/SMX. Current dosages are 300–450 mg of clindamycin every 6 hr and 15 mg of primaquine base once a day for 21 days.

A new drug, atovaquone (Mepron), has been approved on a compassionate basis for the treatment of PCP in patients with HIV disease who cannot tolerate or do not respond to Septra, trimethoprim, dapsone, or parenteral pentamidine. Atovaquone is an oral broad-spectrum antiparasitic drug originally developed to treat malaria. It has shown some activity against PCP. The recommended dosage is 750 mg taken by mouth with food three times a day for 14–21 days. Taking the drug with food is necessary to obtain the appropriate blood levels (AmFAR, Spring 1992b; Howe, 1991c).

Finally, treatment of PCP includes evaluation of ABGs. Oxygenation failure, need for mechanical ventilation, and death are more frequent when marked decreases in ABG levels occur. Administration of corticosteroids with antimicrobial therapy prevents early pulmonary deterioration in patients whose Pa_{O2} is less than 70 mm Hg. The use of corticosteroids also increases exercise tolerance and accelerates recovery. The dosage of prednisone is 40 mg orally twice a day for 5 days followed by 20 mg twice a day for 5 days and then 20 mg each day until the end of antimicrobial therapy (Falloon & Masur, 1992; Montaner et al., 1990). Corticosteroid therapy should be started within 72 hr of antimicrobial therapy.

The effects of antimicrobial therapy on PCP are often slow, and noticeable improvement in ABG levels, findings on chest radiographs, and signs and symptoms may not occur until after 7–10 days of treatment. For this reason, some practitioners switch from treatment with Septra or other oral medications to treatment with pentamidine before 7 or 10 days in an effort to demonstrate improvement.

Careful monitoring of ABGs and pulmonary status are important in order detect respiratory failure early. Despite optimal therapy for PCP, 20% of cases do not respond to initial treatment. Respiratory distress develops, and mechanical ventilation is necessary. Successful treatment and return to breathing without need for mechanical ventilation have been variable. Polis and Masur (1989) reported that of 19 patients on mechanical ventilation for PCP, 42% survived. In another study, 21% survived.

For a mentally competent patient, decisions about intensive care and mechanical ventilation should be made jointly by the patient and the practitioner. The issue should be discussed early in the course of the patient's illness, and all options should be carefully considered. Additional information on this subject is discussed in the chapter on legal and ethical issues.

Drug Side Effects. The most common side effects of treatment with TMP/SMX are nausea and vomiting. Others include fever, rash, neutropenia, thrombocytopenia, and kernicterus. Often patients become intolerant of TMP/SMX as the drug accumulates in the body. Antiemetics are used to control the nausea and vomiting. Diphenhydramine hydrochloride (Benadryl) is used to treat the rash.

The most common side effects of treatment with intravenous pentamidine (Pentam) are neutropenia, hyponatremia, abnormal liver function, and azotemia. Hypoglycemia, orthostatic hypotension, rash, anemia, and facial flushing can also occur. Intramuscular injection of pentamidine can result in local toxic effects, pain, swelling, paresthesia, and sterile abscesses. Muscle loss and paresthesia can persist for months after treatment is completed (Fischl, 1988). Consequently, pentamidine is rarely given intramuscularly.

Hypoglycemia related to treatment with pentamidine can occur as early as 1 hr after the drug is injected and can last up to 7–14 days after treatment is completed. Pentamidine damages islet cells. This causes release of insulin, which produces a hyperinsulin state. Severe hypoglycemia (blood glucose levels of 60 mg/dl or less) can cause seizures and coma.

Medical and nursing management of hypoglycemia is controversial. Generally, blood glucose levels are measured (finger sticks) every 4 hr while the patient is receiving pentamidine intravenously. However, the hypoglycemic effects last long after the drug is stopped. In addition, the glucose level is determined in a random sample of blood (even when done every 4 hr), so a patient's blood glucose level may be lower at any time during the intervals between sampling.

Treatment of hypoglycemia involves administering 50% glucose by intravenous push. This stimulates a rapid increase in the production of insulin, which causes a marked decrease in the blood level of glucose. The result is peaks and valleys rather than a constant level of blood glucose. One way to counteract the effects of pentamidine on blood glucose levels is to have the patient eat foods high in protein and fats and avoid foods high in carbohydrates. Proteins and fat are digested and converted into glucose more slowly than carbohydrates are. A slow release of glucose is more likely to produce a steady blood glucose level.

The side effects of dapsone and trimethoprim are nausea, vomiting, flushing, rash, fever, hemolytic anemia, leukopenia, and hepatotoxic effects. Patients with G6PD deficiency may be at increased risk for hemolytic anemia from dapsone therapy.

The most frequent side effects of treatment with clindamycin are diarrhea and nausea. When clindamycin is used in conjunction with primaquine, the most frequent adverse reaction is rash. Primaquine can also cause hemolysis, especially in patients who have G6PD deficiency.

The most common side effects associated with use of atovaquone are severe rashes, cough, anorexia, nausea, vomiting, diarrhea, fever, headache, constipation, dizziness, and minor blood abnormalities (Falloon & Masur, 1992; Howe, 1991c).

Prophylaxis. Approximately 80% of patients with advanced HIV disease will acquire PCP if they do not have preventive therapy. Of these, 10–25% will not survive (Bartlett, 1992). Consequently, all patients with HIV infection should receive PCP prophylaxis when their CD4 count drops to less than 200 cells/mm^3 (primary prophylaxis) or when they have already had an episode of PCP (secondary prophylaxis). It is currently recommended that patients be started on TMP/SMX (Septra DS) at a dosage of one double-strength tablet each day. The alternative is dapsone 100 mg/day twice a week. If the patient cannot tolerate TMP/SMX or dapsone, aerosolized pentamidine is used.

Prophylaxis with aerosolized pentamidine is used less commonly now because the chance of PCP developing while the patient is taking the medication is 30%, and the relapse rate is even higher. Also, the prevalence of pneumothorax related to PCP is increased because the aerosolized drug does not reach the periphery of the alveoli. In some situations, physicians are prescribing prophylaxis when CD4 counts are less than 300 cells/mm^3 and the percentage of CD4 is less than 20% of the total number of lymphocytes. When aerosolized pentamidine is used for prophylaxis, PCP usually occurs or recurs in the apical areas of the lungs. In order to prevent this, patients should be sitting or turning from side to side if lying down when they receive their pentamidine.

Prophylaxis for PCP has also included use of clindamycin, intravenous pentamidine once or twice a month, and Fansidar. Fansidar is a combination of pyrimethamine (25 mg) and sulfadoxine (500 mg). This drug was initially used as a prophylaxis for travelers in countries where malaria is endemic. Early in the AIDS epidemic, it was used to prevent recurrence of PCP. However, once-a-week dosing is ineffective, and severe, often fatal, skin reactions are common, including erythema multiforme, Stevens-Johnson syndrome, and toxic epidermal neurolysis. Consequently, Fansidar is used only when the patient cannot take alternative drugs (Bartlett, 1992).

Toxoplasma gondii

Toxoplasma gondii is a protozoan. It is the major cause of focal intracerebral lesions in patients with AIDS. The organism is a common pathogen throughout the world. Cats can carry it as oocysts in the gastrointestinal system and eliminate it in the feces. The oocysts can become spores after 24 hr, and the spores can remain in the environment for more than 1 year. The protozoan exists as trophozoites (spores), cysts, and oocysts. The trophozoites invade the cells of the host and multiply, causing cell death and a severe inflammatory response. Trophozoites that survive treatment become encapsulated in cysts.

When a person's immune system is weakened or compromised, the cell wall of the cysts can break down, releasing trophozoites to infect other areas of the body (Fahrner & Nelson, 1988).

Toxoplasma gondii is transmitted by contact with contaminated cat feces or by ingestion of raw or undercooked meat from infected cattle, lambs, or swine. In humans, infection with toxoplasmal spores usually causes a respiratory illness, which may not be symptomatic. The most common site of infection is the central nervous system. The second most common site is the lung. Infection of the heart, peritoneum, skin, and colon can also occur (Sande & Volberding, 1992). Studies are being done to determine if infants born to women with toxoplasmosis are at increased risk for congenital toxoplasmosis.

Signs and Symptoms. The signs and symptoms of toxoplasmosis may be vague and nonspecific. Patients may have fever or headaches. They could also have nausea, vomiting, lethargy, and malaise. Some patients have meningeal and focal neurologic signs and symptoms or experience seizures. Patients with toxoplasmic encephalitis may have fever or headache. Up to 60% have altered mental status, which is seen as confusion, lethargy, cognitive impairment, or coma (Sande & Volberding, 1992).

Diagnostic Evaluation. Diagnosis is based on biopsy findings. Specimens of the lesion(s) or stains of spinal fluid show the typical spores. Spinal fluid also has increased numbers of white cells and increased levels of protein. CT scans obtained after injection of contrast material show a ring-enhancing lesion or multiple lesions. The level of antibodies to *Toxoplasma* is usually quite elevated.

Biopsy of the lesions is associated with high morbidity and mortality. Therefore, most physicians follow progress of therapy for 2–3 weeks. They obtain additional CT scans of the head and look for shrinkage of the lesion or lesions. Repeated lumbar punctures are not helpful except to eliminate other causes of illness when therapy appears to be ineffective.

Treatment. Treatment begins with a loading dose of pyrimethamine (100–200 mg). This is followed by 6 weeks of pyrimethamine (50–100 mg/day), sulfadiazine (1 g four times a day), and folinic acid (5–10 mg/day). Folinic acid prevents decreases in the WBC. Clindamycin is sometimes used in place of sulfadiazine. Azithromycin is used for patients who do not respond to or cannot tolerate the standard treatment.

There is no cure for toxoplasmosis. The spores can be eradicated, but the cysts cannot. Patients who are immunocompromised can be reinfected. Lifelong suppressive therapy is necessary to prevent this. The current recommended regimen for suppressive therapy is a combination of pyrimethamine, folinic acid, and sulfadiazine (Bartlett, 1992).

Finally, some retrospective data suggest that PCP prophylaxis with Septra or dapsone also prevents toxoplasmosis. Further information on the effectiveness of Septra or dapsone for prophylaxis of toxoplasmosis will be available in the future.

Drug Side Effects. Pyrimethamine is often associated with a macular, papular, erythematous, pruritic rash. Nausea, vomiting, and diarrhea are also common. Blood counts should be monitored on a regular basis because pancytopenia may occur.

The side effects of sulfadiazine are similar to those caused by other sulfa drugs. These include rash, pancytopenia, nausea, vomiting, and diarrhea. Azithromycin causes nausea, vomiting, diarrhea, hepatic toxic effects, indigestion, flatulence, headache, and dizziness.

For information on the side of clindamycin, see the section on PCP.

Cryptosporidium

Cryptosporidium is a genus of intestinal protozoa that causes severe watery diarrhea. The volume of fluid lost is tremendous, up to 4 quarts/day. In immunocompetent persons, the infection is a self-limiting. The diarrhea lasts 4–20 days.

Signs and Symptoms. In addition to severe diarrhea, cryptosporidiosis causes malaise, nausea, and abdominal cramping. The large volumes of fluid lost can cause depletion of sodium, potassium, and chloride. Prolonged diarrhea results in severe weight loss, malnutrition, and debilitation.

Diagnostic Evaluation. The diagnosis is based on showing the presence of the oocyst in the stool. Modified acid-fast stains of stool smears are used.

Treatment. Currently, no effective treatment of cryptosporidiosis is available. The usual antiprotozoal drugs and antidiarrheal agents are ineffective. Care should include supportive measures such as adequate hydration, nutritional supplements, and antidiarrheal agents such as Lomotil or paregoric. Enteric precautions should be used, because the organisms can be transmitted through contact with contaminated waste.

Fungal Opportunistic Infections

Candida albicans

Candida albicans is the cause of the most frequent fungal infection in patients with HIV disease. It does not affect mortality, but it does increase morbidity. *Candida* primarily causes severe infections in the mouth and esophagus. It may also affect the skin, nails, urinary tract, vagina, and the lower part of the gastrointestinal tract. The organism is disseminated by the bloodstream. Consequently, it is sometimes found on heart structures and in the blood. It is often found in the respiratory tract. Its presence in sputum or bronchial washings is not uncommon. *Candida* is part of the normal microbial flora, and small quantities do not indicate a significant infection. *Candida* esophagitis is an AIDS-defining condition.

Candidiasis occurs because of a reduction in the normal bacterial flora (as from antibiotic therapy) or an imbalance in hormonal or nutritional status. It also occurs when the skin or mucosal barriers are disrupted or cell-mediated immunity is impaired (Newlin & Stringari, 1988). In persons with HIV infection, it is seen when CD4 counts are higher than 500 cells/mm^3. *Candida* is considered a pathogen only when it overgrows other microorganisms or causes tissue damage.

Oral candidiasis (thrush) and *Candida* esophagitis can be severe infections in persons with HIV disease. Thrush may be the first opportunistic infection in this population.

Vaginal candidiasis is the most common initial clinical manifestation of HIV infection in women. It occurs throughout the spectrum of HIV disease. Although the infection usually responds to clotrimazole (Gyne-Lotrimin), it frequently recurs. Persistent candidiasis may require treatment with fluconazole or amphotericin B (Bartlett, 1992; Wofsy, 1992).

Signs and Symptoms. Severe oral candidiasis is characterized by sore throat, mouth, or tongue; foul taste; and white patches on the tongue, throat, hard palate, or buccal mucosa. Candida esophagitis is characterized by difficulty swallowing (dysphagia), severe pain when swallowing (odynophagia), and white patches in the esophagus. Vaginal candidiasis causes burning and itching in the pubic and vaginal areas and is associated with a thick, white, cottage cheese–like, foul-smelling vaginal discharge. Skin lesions are discolored flat areas with irregular dry white scaling borders. These lesions cause itching, redness, and maceration of moist areas. Candida is frequently the culprit in athlete's foot, jock itch, and many infections of the skin on the trunk and extremities.

Diagnostic Evaluation. Oral candidiasis is usually diagnosed on the basis of the white patches it causes. It can also be detected by microscopic examination of scrapings of the patches or by culture of the fungus from samples taken from the mucous membranes. The scrapings are treated with potassium hydroxide, and special medium is used for culture. Radiographs of the upper part of the gastrointestinal tract or endoscopy with biopsy and culture are used to diagnose *Candida* esophagitis. Systemic infections are detected by growing the agent from biopsy specimens of the affected organ or from blood.

Treatment. Oral candidiasis is treated with topical medications. Nystatin (Nilstat) liquid, 500,000 U/5 ml four times a day, used as a swish and swallow; clotrimazole (Mycelex) troches, 10 mg; or nystatin vaginal tablets dissolved in the mouth one to five times a day (Greenspan, Greenspan, & Winkler, 1990) may be used. Oral ketoconazole (Nizoril), 200–400 mg/day for 5–7 days is the medication of choice for treatment of the initial infection. Once the obvious infection has resolved, use of clotrimazole or nystatin one or two times a day helps prevent recurrence.

Fluconazole is also being used to treat oral candidiasis that has become resistant to clotrimazole and ketoconazole. The usual dosage is 50–100 mg/day for 7–21 days. If the infection recurs after this regimen, the patient is treated again and then started on suppressive therapy with fluconazole at a dosage of 100 mg/day.

Candida esophagitis is best treated with ketoconazole, 200–400 mg twice a day for 7–14 days or until signs and symptoms have been resolved for more than a week. If signs and symptoms recur, treatment is repeated, and then a regimen of 100–200 mg/day is started as suppressive therapy. Continued use of ketoconazole is not recommended unless the infection recurs after suppressive therapy with nystatin or clotrimazole because of the effect of the drug on the liver. In addition, ketoconazole requires an acid environment for absorption and effective response. Therefore, patients should take the drug with orange juice or grapefruit juice and cannot be taking cimetidine (Tagamet) or antacids.

When clotrimazole, nystatin, ketoconazole, and fluconazole are ineffective in treatment of oral or esophageal candidiasis, intravenous amphotericin B, 0.25–1.5 mg/kg per day, has been used. After 5–7 days of treatment, oral nystatin or amphotericin B may be used. Oral amphotericin B is usually given once or twice a week.

Cutaneous candidiasis usually responds to treatment with over-the-counter antifungal agents, such as clotrimazole cream or lotion or nystatin cream. Occasionally, creams that contain cortisone are needed to treat both the fungus and the inflammation caused by the fungus.

Vaginal candidiasis is treated with Gyne-Lotrimin cream or tablets inserted into the vaginal vault twice a day for 7 days. If treatment with topical agents is ineffective, oral ketoconazole, 200 mg/day for 5–7 days, is used (Bartlett, 1992). Persistent infection may require treatment with fluconazole or amphotericin B (Wofsy, 1992).

Drug Side Effects. Clotrimazole troches and nystatin suspension may leave a foul taste in the mouth. Occasionally, treatment with this drug causes increased levels of liver enzymes. Clotrimazole vaginal cream or tablets can cause rash, burning, blistering, and peeling.

Ketoconazole may cause increases in the level of liver enzymes. For this reason, long-term use of the drug is usually avoided. Ketoconazole can also cause gynecomastia, diarrhea, nausea and vomiting, and adrenal suppression.

For information on the side effects of fluconazole and amphotericin B, see the following section on cryptococcal infections.

Sources: Crocker, 1989; Newlin & Stringari, 1988; Pape, 1988.

Cryptococcus neoformans

Cryptococcus neoformans is the most common cause of fungal meningitis and disseminated disease in patients who are immunocompromised. It is the fourth most common opportunistic infection in HIV-infected persons. The primary sites of infection are the central nervous system and blood. The organism can also infect the lungs, heart, gastrointestinal tract, bone, prostate, eye, skin, and lymphatic system.

The fungus is found worldwide in the soil and in pigeon droppings. Its point of entry is the lungs. In immunocompetent persons, *C. neoformans* causes an asymptomatic infection. Patients who are immunocompromised have severe infections because their T lymphocytes and macrophages cannot destroy the organism. In these patients, fungi in the lung frequently enter the bloodstream and are carried to other organs. The fungi are probably transported to the central nervous system by macrophages or monocytes.

Signs and Symptoms. The clinical features of cryptococcal infections are usually vague and nonspecific. Patients' complaints range from fever, headache, and malaise to nausea, photophobia, and alteration in mental status (Sande & Volberding, 1992). The infection becomes disseminated in most patients. Fungus in the bloodstream (fungemia) is characterized by fever, nausea, vomiting, and fatigue. Blood cultures are positive for *Cryptococcus,* and cryptococcal antigens can be detected in the serum.

Diagnostic Evaluation. Diagnosis is based on detection of increased levels of cryptococcal antigen in serum or cerebrospinal fluid. Analysis of cerebrospinal fluid will show increased levels of protein and white cells and decreased levels of glucose. Staining with India ink will show encapsulated cryptococci.

Treatment. The standard treatment is amphotericin B with or without 5-flucytosine (5FC). However, the side effects of these drugs are severe. Therefore, fluconazole (Diflucan) is being used as a practical alternative. Fluconazole can cross the blood-brain barrier and has minimal side effects. Treatment with fluconazole reduces the levels of cryptococcal antigen in the serum and cerebrospinal fluid. In some situations, patients are being started on 400 mg/day by mouth. After treatment for 6 weeks, the dosage is reduced to 200 mg/day. This dosage is continued unless a persistent increase in the level of cryptococcal antigen occurs.

Amphotericin B is administered over 3–4 hr by infusion through a central venous access line such as a Hickman or Groshong catheter. A central venous catheter is used to prevent thrombophlebitis at the peripheral intravenous site. The dosage is 0.3–1.0 mg/kg per day. Initial doses are very low. The dosage is increased slowly until the optimum daily dose is reached. The slow increase is used to detect intolerance to the drug and to prevent renal toxic effects. Once patients tolerate daily doses, treatment may be modified to three times a week to prevent possible damage to the kidneys. A total of 1–2 g of the drug is administered.

Infusion of amphotericin B frequently causes severe fevers and shaking chills (rigors). In order to prevent these side effects, patients are given 50 mg of diphenhydramine hydrochloride and 650 mg of acetaminophen 30 min before infusion of amphotericin B begins. In addition, 25–50 mg of hydrocortisone is added to the amphotericin to reduce the occurrence of rigors, and 50–100 mg of meperidine is used to treat severe rigors.

In addition to amphotericin B, flucytosine is given orally at 150 mg/kg per day in four divided doses. Frequent spinal taps and determination of antigen levels are required to monitor progress and the effectiveness of treatment. When flucytosine is used as the sole treatment, development of drug-resistant organisms is rapid. Consequently, it is rarely used alone.

Preliminary studies on the effectiveness of fluconazole have had encouraging results. Treatment with this drug improves the overall course of cryptococcal infections. Prolonged hospitalization is not needed, and the risk of bacteremia from infection of a central venous line or catheter is eliminated. In addition, fluconazole does not cause depletion of potassium, magnesium, or phosphate ("FDA Notes," 1990).

Drug Side Effects. The primary side effect of amphotericin B is reversible impairment of renal function. Serum levels of blood urea nitrogen (BUN) and creatinine should be monitored closely. The dosage of amphotericin B should be changed if the level of creatinine is more than 2.5–3.0/dl.

Amphotericin B also decreases the levels of magnesium, potassium, and phosphate in the blood. When this occurs, intravenous administration of 1–4 g of magnesium before the amphotericin is infused will replace the magnesium and potentially increase the level of phosphate. Potassium is replaced orally. Intravenous administration of high doses of potassium requires cardiac monitoring because of possible arrhythmias. Potassium chloride can be given safely intravenously if the rate is no higher than 10 mEq/hr.

Rash is the most common side effect of treatment with flucytosine. Patients may also experience gastrointestinal intolerance, hepatitis, and bone marrow suppression with associated anemia and leukopenia.

The primary side effects of fluconazole are nausea, vomiting, and diarrhea. All these are manageable and are more tolerable than the side effects associated with infusion of amphotericin B.

Prophylaxis. Like most opportunistic infections, cryptococcosis often recurs. In the past, amphotericin B twice a week was used to prevent relapses. Currently, fluconazole, 200-400 mg/day orally, is recommended for maintenance therapy. Other oral drugs such as ketoconazole and itraconazole have not been effective in preventing relapses (Tozzi et al., 1989).

Sources: Grant & Armstrong, 1988; Newlin & Stringari, 1988; Wolfe, 1989.

Histoplasma capsulatum

Histoplasmosis is another fungal blood infection that occurs more often now in patients with HIV infection. The disease is endemic in the central and south-central states in the United States, and in Mexico and the Caribbean. The causative agent, *Histoplasma capsulatum,* is found in soil heavily contaminated with bird or bat droppings. It may also be found in chicken coops and grain silos.

Histoplasmosis occurs in those who have lived or traveled in an endemic area. In persons with a healthy immune system, the disease is usually asymptomatic and self-limiting. In patients who are immunocompromised, histoplasmosis is a disseminated infection. It may be the first manifestation of AIDS, or it may be associated with other opportunistic infections. Reactivation of latent disease occurs in some patients (Kovacs & Masur, 1988). *Histoplasma* spores are inhaled into the respiratory tract. From there, they enter the bloodstream. Once in the bloodstream. they spread rapidly to the bone marrow, liver, spleen, lymph nodes, and cerebrospinal fluid.

Signs and Symptoms. Histoplasmosis is characterized by fever, chills, sweats, nausea, vomiting, diarrhea, weight loss, and severe fatigue. The presence of a cough may indicate a pneumonitis, which is seen as a diffuse, patchy, reticulonodular infiltrate on chest radiographs. Caseating (cheeselike) or noncaseating granulomas may occur.

Diagnostic Evaluation. The most common methods of diagnosis are detection of *H. capsulatum* in bone marrow smears and growth of the fungus in blood and sputum cultures. Serologic tests for *Histoplasma* and detection of the organism in biopsy specimens of lymph nodes are also used. Patients may have increased levels of liver enzymes, neutropenia, thrombocytopenia, and an enlarged liver.

Treatment. Amphotericin B, 0.5–1.0 mg/kg per day for 4–8 weeks for a total of 1.0–2.5 g, is the treatment of choice. Suppressive therapy is required to prevent relapses. Amphotericin B is usually used. In preliminary studies, itraconazole, an experimental drug, was effective in suppressing recurrence. Ketoconazole is not effective for either initial treatment or maintenance therapy (Sande & Volberding, 1992).

Drug Side Effects. For information on the side effects of amphotericin B and ketoconazole, see the section on cryptococcal infections. The side effects of treatment with itraconazole are nausea and increased levels of liver enzymes.

Sources: Minamoto & Armstrong, 1988; Newlin & Stringari, 1988.

Coccidioides immitis

Coccidioidomycosis is widespread in central California, Arizona, and Mexico. It also can be found in the southwestern United States, from Texas to California. It is usually a pulmonary infection, but it may cause disseminated disease. The causative agent is *Coccidioides immitis.* Spores of the fungus are found in the soil. Infection occurs when the spores are inhaled. In persons with HIV infection, coccidioidomycosis rarely occurs when the CD4 count is greater than 250 cells/mm^3.

Signs and Symptoms. In patients who are immunocompromised, the signs and symptoms of coccidioidomycosis are severe shortness of breath, fever, and anorexia.

Diagnostic Evaluation. In cases of pulmonary coccidioidomycosis, chest radiographs show cavitary lesions throughout the lungs. Patients may or may not react to skin tests for *Coccidioides*. If the immunosuppression is severe, the patient may be anergic. In disseminated disease, the fungus can be detected in blood cultures, bone marrow aspirates, and tissue samples. Serologic tests for *Coccidioides* will be positive.

Treatment. Like other fungal infections, coccidioidomycosis is treated with amphotericin B. The dosage is 0.5–1.0 mg/kg per day intravenously for 4–8 weeks for a total of 1.0–2.5 g. After initial treatment, suppressive therapy is required to prevent relapse. Either amphotericin B or fluconazole is used.

Drug Side Effects. For information on the side effects of amphotericin B and fluconazole, see the section on cryptococcal infections.

Sources: Minamoto & Armstrong, 1988; Newlin & Stringari, 1988.

Bacterial Infections

Mycobacterium tuberculosis

Tuberculosis caused by *Mycobacterium tuberculosis* (MTB) is becoming more common in persons infected with HIV. Since 1984, the prevalence of tuberculosis in the United States has increased markedly. Much of the increase has been attributed to HIV infection. In addition, multidrug-resistant strains of MTB have developed.

In the general population, the prevalence of MTB infection is high among drug users and among persons who live in economically deprived or less technologically developed areas. Probably, reactivation of latent primary disease occurs and is more frequent in persons who have progressive T-cell depression.

Mycobacterium tuberculosis is a slow-growing, thin, rod-shaped, obligate aerobe. It is transmitted from person to person by aerosolized droplets. The presence of MTB in HIV-infected individuals is secondary to the loss of cellular immunity, which normally promotes host resistance. One half to two-thirds of MTB infections involve sites outside the lungs. The most common of these are peripheral lymph nodes and bone marrow (Sande & Volberding, 1992). MTB tuberculosis often occurs concurrently with other opportunistic diseases, such as PCP or Kaposi's sarcoma.

Signs and Symptoms. The signs and symptoms of MTB tuberculosis are fever, severe night sweats, cough, and shortness of breath. Disseminated infection is characterized by fever, chills, sweats, nausea, vomiting, weight loss, and debilitation. Involvement of the central nervous system may cause headache, confusion or changes in mental status, fever, chills, and sweats. Gastrointestinal involvement is characterized by nausea, vomiting, diarrhea, and abdominal pain.

Diagnostic Evaluation. In cases of active pulmonary tuberculosis, chest radiographs show diffuse pulmonary infiltrates, mostly in the upper lobes of the lungs, or focal consolidation with or without cavitation. Intrathoracic adenopathy or pleural effusions occur in 25% of patients.

Anergy is common among patients who are seropositive for HIV. Only 10–40% of these patients have positive reactions to skin tests with purified protein derivative (PPD) at the time tuberculosis is diagnosed (Sande & Volberding, 1992). All patients who are suspected of having tuberculosis should be screened. A negative skin test does not mean MTB is not present. If the quantity of MTB in sputum is sufficient, the organism can be seen on smears. It can also be cultured from blood, cerebrospinal fluid, or biopsy specimens. In cases of spinal tuberculosis, analysis of cerebrospinal fluid will show a decrease in the level of glucose, increases in the level of protein and the number of white cells, and the presence of acid-fast bacilli.

Treatment. The CDC recommends a combination of drugs. Oral doses of isoniazid (300 mg), rifampin (600 mg), and pyrazinamide (20–30 mg/kg) are taken daily for the first 2 months. Isoniazid, rifampin, and pyridoxine (vitamin B$_6$) are taken for the next 7 months. Pyridoxine, 50 mg/day orally, is given to prevent potential neurologic symptoms. If multidrug-resistant MTB is suspected, a fourth medication, usually ethambutol (15–25 mg/kg per day), is added. It is given for the entire 9 months of treatment.

Drug Side Effects. The most common side effects are gastrointestinal. Isoniazid can cause hepatitis, fever, rash, and peripheral neuropathy. Because of the frequency of hepatitis, liver function tests should be done before treatment with isoniazid is started, and levels of liver enzymes should be monitored closely during treatment.

Rifampin can cause nausea, vomiting, rash, flulike symptoms, thrombocytopenia, and jaundice. It can also cause color blindness, so color vision should be checked on a regular basis. Patients should also be told that their urine and other body fluids may turn orange. Rifampin also increases the metabolism of dapsone, fluconazole, ketoconazole, methadone, oral contraceptives, corticosteroids, and sulfonylureas. When rifampin is given in conjunction with methadone, it may precipitate signs and symptoms of acute methadone withdrawal (Amodio-Groton, 1992).

Pyrazinamide causes hepatitis, nausea, vomiting, dysuria, malaise, anorexia, arthralgia, and fever. Dementia, pruritus, joint pain, gastrointestinal upset, abdominal pain, fever, malaise, headache, dizziness, and changes in mental status may occur with ethambutol.

PPD Converters. The risk of tuberculosis developing is high for persons who are seropositive for HIV. They should have skin tests with PPD every 6 months. Tests with control antigens, such as those for *Candida* and mumps virus, should be included to determine anergy. Patients whose reactions change from negative to positive for PPD should have a chest radiograph and start chemoprophylaxis with isoniazid at a dosage of 300 mg/day. The length of treatment is still controversial. However, PPD converters who are immunocompetent usually take isoniazid for 9–12 months. Some practitioners have proposed lifelong prophylaxis for PPD converters who are immunosuppressed. Finally, those with positive PPD tests whose previous status is unknown should also be treated with isoniazid (Chaisson & Slutkin, 1989).

Sources: Carr & Marin, 1988; Kovacs & Masur, 1988; Polis & Masur, 1989.

Mycobacterium avium-intracellulare

Mycobacterium avium-intracellulare (MAI) or *Mycobacterium avium* complex (MAC) is a common bacterium found in the environment. It is the second most common species of potentially pathogenic *Mycobacterium*. It rarely causes infection in persons who have healthy immune systems. In persons who are seropositive for HIV, disseminated infection with MAI usually occurs later in the HIV disease process. Often, the infection is not detected before autopsy (Bartlett, Laughon, & Quinn, 1988; Pitchenik, 1988). Infection with MAI is slowly progressive, but it is rarely the cause of death. However, the severe signs and symptoms leave the patient weak and extremely fatigued and eventually interfere with the quality of life.

MAI infection is acquired by ingesting or inhaling the bacterium. The organism disseminates rapidly throughout the body. The liver, spleen, lymph nodes, bone marrow, and gastrointestinal tract may be infected (Flaskerud & Ungvarski, 1992).

Signs and Symptoms. The signs and symptoms are generally vague, nonspecific, and consistent with systemic infection. They include fever, fatigue, weight loss, diarrhea, and night sweats. In disseminated infections, anemia, leukopenia, and thrombocytopenia may occur. Respiratory signs and symptoms are rare.

Diagnostic Evaluation. Diagnosis of MAI infection is based on detection of the bacterium in cultures of sputum, stool, tissue, or blood. Many months may pass before the number of organisms present is high enough for identification.

Treatment. Treatment of MAI infection is difficult because the organism is often resistant to drugs. No single drug or combination of drugs has shown reliable antimicrobial activity. Patients with minimal signs and symptoms usually are not treated because the drugs used have severe side effects. Patients with severe signs and symptoms may benefit from treatment, which may decrease or alleviate the signs and symptoms. In these cases, management of the drugs' gastrointestinal side effects is a major problem.

Combinations of the following drugs have been used to treat MAI infections:

> Isoniazid (INH), 300 mg/day orally (if infection with *M. tuberculosis* is considered likely)
> Rifampin (Rifadin, Rifampicin), 600 mg/day orally
> Ethambutol (Myambutol), 800–1200 mg/day (or 25 mg/kg per day) orally
> Clofazamine (Lamprene), 100–200 mg/day orally
> Amikacin (Amikin), 7.5 mg/kg twice a day or 10 mg/kg once a day intramuscularly or intravenously
> Ciprofloxacin, 500–750 mg twice a day orally
> Rifabutin (Ansamycin), 300 mg/day orally
> Clarithromycin (Biaxin), 500–900 mg twice a day orally

Most often treatment includes a combination of ciprofloxacin, ethambutol, clofazamine, and rifampin. Recently, clarithromycin has been used in combination with ethambutol (Chaisson, McCuthan, Nightengale, & Young, 1993). The combination is used because MAI appears to become resistant to clarithromycin after 3 months when this drug is used alone. Although long-term data are not available, patients have reported decreases in fever, sweats, fatigue, and weight loss and an overall improvement in the quality of life. Azithromycin (Zithromax) also has been used for treatment, and rifabutin has been used for prophylaxis (AmFAR, Spring 1992c).

The side effects from the combination of drugs can be severe. The gastrointestinal ones are the most significant. Management of nausea, vomiting, diarrhea, and dehydration is important, and hospitalization may be necessary. The gastrointestinal distress may be reduced if the drugs are started one at a time, with slow addition of each new drug.

Drug Side Effects. The side effects of treatment with isoniazid, rifampin, and ethambutol are discussed in the section on MTB. The side effect of clofazamine is hyperpigmentation. The skin may become very dark. This is not harmful to the patient's well-being.

Clarithromycin causes nausea, vomiting, diarrhea, rash, hepatotoxic effects, heartburn, anorexia, and headache. Rifabutin can cause an increase in the levels of liver enzymes and a decrease in the number of platelets. It also makes the urine turn red-orange and increases the metabolism of other drugs, such as rifampin. Rifabutin and rifampin should not be used together.

Amikacin can cause irritation at the site of injection, increases in the levels of liver enzymes, pancytopenia, and nephrotoxic effects. Use of ciprofloxacin is associated with rash, nausea, vomiting, leukopenia, and anemia.

The side effects of azithromycin are discussed in the section on protozoal infections.

Sources: Bartlett et al., 1988; Carr & Marin, 1988; Chaisson & Slutkin, 1989; Hoy et al., 1990; O'Grady & Frasier, 1992; Pitchenik, 1988; and Polis & Masur, 1989.

Staphylococcus aureus

Staphylococcus aureus is a gram-positive aerobic bacterium that grows in clusters. It is part of the normal flora. All humans have this bacterium on their skin and in their mouth and nose. In immunocompromised patients, the frequency of local skin infections and bacteremia due to *S. aureus* is high. These infections are more common in drug users. Treatment of staphylococcal infections can be difficult if drug-resistant strains develop. Infections due to methicillin-resistant *S. aureus* are becoming more common.

Signs and Symptoms. Skin infections caused by *S. aureus* are characterized by redness, warmth, pain, and induration. If these infections are not treated promptly and appropriately, abscesses or lymphangitis can develop.

Bacteremia causes fever (body temperature as high as 104°F [40°C]), chills, rigors, sweats, headache, arthralgia, myalgia, hypotension, lethargy, and confusion. Signs and symptoms of shock may also be evident.

One complication of severe bacteremia is the development of staphylococcal emboli. They often appear as small black or purple pinpoint areas on the tips of the fingers or toes or as larger areas that cover the entire finger, toe, foot, arm, or leg. The emboli may also affect the bowel, lungs, liver, heart, and brain. Another complication of bacteremia is the development of staphylococcal abscesses in the liver, spleen, lung, and brain. Endocarditis and cardiac valve disease are also possible. Endocarditis is an important complication of staphylococcal infection related to use of intravenous drugs.

Diagnostic Evaluation. Diagnosis is based on detecting the organism in material taken from the site of infection. Microscopic examination of smears of exudates from lesions will show clusters of gram-positive cocci. Blood smears will also show the organisms.

Treatment. Localized infections are treated with dicloxacillin sodium, 500 mg four times a day for 10–14 days. Patients allergic to penicillin-related drugs can be given ciprofloxacin, 250 mg four times a day for 10–14 days.

Bacteremia and endocarditis are treated with intravenous penicillin four times a day for 6 weeks. Patients allergic to penicillin may receive a cephalosporin derivative or vancomycin hydrochloride.

Drug Side Effects. The most common side effects for all these drugs are rash, fever, changes in the levels of liver enzymes, renal damage, and development of bacterial resistance to the drug.

Sources: Pitchenik, 1988; Polis & Masur, 1989.

Salmonella Species

Salmonellosis is a bacterial infection caused by gram-negative rods. The organisms are transmitted by the fecal-oral route. Humans usually acquire the infection by eating or drinking food products contaminated with the bacteria. In patients infected with HIV, infection with *Salmonella* often causes bacteremia. Recurrent salmonellosis in a person infected with HIV is an AIDS-defining condition.

Salmonella is a common organism. It is found in chicken, fish, eggs, and unpasteurized milk and milk products. Patients with HIV disease should not add raw eggs to milk or other drinks to increase the drinks' caloric content. They should not eat undercooked chicken or raw fish as in sushi or ceviche. They should avoid unpasteurized milk and products, such as cheese and yogurt, made from unpasteurized milk.

Signs and Symptoms. Gastrointestinal *Salmonella* infections cause severe diarrhea and abdominal cramping. Occasionally, blood and mucus may be seen in the feces. *Salmonella* bacteremia causes fever and shaking chills, malaise, fatigue, anorexia, cachexia, myalgia, and weight loss. These may be preceded by gastrointestinal signs and symptoms.

Diagnostic Evaluation. Diagnosis is based on culture of *Salmonella* from blood or stool samples. Occasionally, a history of eating raw eggs or unpasteurized milk or of foreign travel will provide a clue to the diagnosis.

Treatment. The most common agent used to treat diarrhea caused by *Salmonella* is ampicillin, 500 mg orally four times a day for 7–10 days. Other drugs that may be used include TMP/SMX (Septra), usually at double strength, twice a day for 7–10 days; cephtriaxone (Rocephin); and ciprofloxacin.

Initial treatment of bacteremia is intravenous ampicillin or Septra. Both the diarrhea and the bacteremia may recur or become chronic. Suppressive treatment with ampicillin or Septra may be used to prevent this.

Drug Side Effects. The major side effects of ampicillin are rash and other allergic manifestations. Allergic reactions such as rash and fever may also occur with Septra. Both ampicillin and Septra may cause nausea, vomiting, and diarrhea.

Sources: Bartlett et al., 1988; Crocker, 1989.

Shigella Species

Shigellosis is a gastrointestinal infection caused by gram-negative bacteria. The organisms can be transmitted from one person to another by the fecal-oral route. *Shigella* species are also found in contaminated water supplies and in shellfish in some areas of the world. *Shigella* rarely cause bacteremia in persons infected with HIV.

Signs and Symptoms. The major signs and symptoms are liquid stool containing blood and mucus and abdominal cramps that increase in severity just before defecation. Fever and chills are also present.

Diagnostic Evaluation. Diagnosis is based on detection of the bacterium in cultures of stool samples. Microscopic examination of stool samples will show many white blood cells, indicating an inflammatory process.

Treatment. The most common drugs used to treat shigellosis are oral ampicillin, 500 mg four times a day, and oral Septra, double strength twice a day. Ciprofloxacin, 500 mg four times a day, may also be used.

Drug Side Effects. The side effects of these three drugs are described in previous sections.

Sources: Bartlett et al., 1988; Crocker, 1989.

Viral Opportunistic Infections

The presence and recurrence of opportunistic viral infections in persons infected with HIV are common. The ones seen most often are caused by herpes simplex virus types 1 and 2 (HSV-1 and HSV-2, respectively), varicella-zoster virus (VZV), and cytomegalovirus (CMV). Table 13 gives general treatments for these infections.

Herpes Simplex Virus

Herpes simplex viruses are DNA viruses. Both HSV-1 and HSV-2 are common in the general population. They are responsible for considerable morbidity in patients with HIV disease. Many adults with AIDS were exposed to HSV before they became infected with HIV. Therefore, they are not susceptible to primary infection with HSV (Sande & Volberding,

1992). Recurrent HSV infections are more common than primary infections.

In persons with a healthy immune system, recurrences of HSV-1 infection can be brought on by illness, stress, or exposure to the sun. HSV-2 causes genital and perineal ulcerations and is sexually transmitted. In persons infected with HIV, HSV-2 has been associated with painful perianal ulcerations, proctitis, and vaginitis. Occasionally, HSV-2 is found in the mouth or the facial area around the mouth.

Signs and Symptoms. HSV-1 causes benign ulcers of the nose, mouth, pharynx, esophagus, and skin. The ulcers have an erythematous base and a white center. The most common complaint is burning pain at the site of the lesion. Esophageal ulcers cause severe dysphagia and odynophagia. Severe oral ulcerations may be confused with aphthous ulcers, which do not respond to treatment with acyclovir.

HSV-2 causes burning, painful ulcerations that initially appear as singular, small, blisterlike eruptions. The ulcerations may coalesce on the genital, perineal, and perianal areas. Perianal ulcers are frequently described as hemorrhoids, with or without bleeding. Perianal and rectal infections cause bleeding, tenesmus, and bowel or urinary problems. The bowel and bladder problems may be due to the proximity and involvement of the sacral plexus, which also may become infected with the virus. Before treatment with acyclovir was available, severe ulcerations and erosion of the perianal and rectal areas often occurred. Sometimes these erosions were so severe that they prevented normal bowel movements, and superimposed infections occurred. Colostomies were necessary for healing.

Diagnostic Evaluation. Diagnosis is based primarily on the appearance of the lesions. The viruses can be cultured from scrapings of the lesions. A special viral culture medium is required.

Treatment. Acyclovir (Zovirax) is recommended for treatment of HSV infections. It is used for severe HSV-1 infections of the mouth, face, pharynx, and esophagus. It is also used to treat perianal, perineal, and genital infections and to prevent recurrent infections. The dosage for initial treatment of mild infections causing mouth, perianal, or genital ulcers is 200 mg orally five times a day. HSV esophagitis and severe perianal and rectal herpes infections should be treated with intravenous acyclovir for 7 days. Maintenance therapy is 200 mg two to three times a day orally.

Foscarnet (Foscavir) has been used to treat acyclovir-resistant HSV. Foscarnet is given intravenously. The initial dosage is 40–60 mg/kg every 8 hr given over 2 hr for 2–3 weeks. If the HSV infection resolves, no further treatment may be required. If a response occurs, but the infection does not resolve, foscarnet may be continued as a daily regimen.

The major problem with foscarnet is that it irritates the vein. A central line and a pump or controller are required to control the rate of infusion. If the drug is given through a peripheral line, it is diluted by adding 250–500 ml of saline. The drug is now dispensed in 250- or 500-ml glass bottles containing foscarnet at a concentration of 24 mg/ml.

Foscarnet is also quite damaging to the kidneys. The dosage is adjusted for patients with decreased creatinine clearance. Finally, in order to reduce the potential renal toxic effects and to maintain hydration, 1,000 ml of saline is given along with one dose each day or before or after a daily dose.

Drug Side Effects. Acyclovir is well tolerated orally. Side effects are usually renal effects, such as elevated levels of BUN and creatinine. Renal toxic effects can be prevented by maintaining hydration.

Side effects caused by foscarnet are nausea, vomiting, hypokalemia, hypomagnesemia, hypocalcemia, and hypophosphatemia. More serious effects, such as

CHAPTER 7 — MEDICAL MANAGEMENT OF OPPORTUNISTIC INFECTIONS, TUMORS, AND AIDS DEMENTIA COMPLEX

frank tetany, seizures, and arrhythmias, may be related to imbalances in electrolytes and minerals. Serum levels of potassium, magnesium, calcium, phosphate, BUN, and creatinine should be determined at least once or twice a week. If the creatinine clearance rate increases, the dose of foscarnet should be changed. The manufacturer, Astra Pharmaceutical Products, Inc., has developed a dosing schedule for patients who have increases in creatinine clearance.

Sources: Bartlett et al., 1988; Crumpacker, 1988; Drew et al., 1988; Feinberg, 1992; O'Dell & Zender, 1988; Polis & Masur, 1989.

Herpes Zoster or Varicella-Zoster Virus

Varicella-zoster virus (VZV) is a herpesvirus. It is best known as the cause of chickenpox and shingles. The acute primary infection (varicella or chickenpox) usually occurs during childhood. It is self-limiting in children with competent immune systems. In adults, however, primary infection can be severe. The virus is easily transmitted by direct contact with infectious lesions or by inhalation of aerosolized infected droplets. Transmission can occur 1–2 days before the onset of rash and lasts until the lesions are dried (Cohen, Sande, & Volberding, 1990). Complications are common in immunocompromised patients and may cause prolonged morbidity or death. Varicella pneumonia and varicella encephalitis have been reported.

Recurrent VZV infection (zoster or shingles) may occur because of a weakened immune system. Recurrence is common in the general population. After the initial episode of chickenpox, the virus migrates and becomes latent in the sensory ganglia. During times of stress, other infections, surgery, or immunosuppression, the virus can be reactivated. It then travels down the sensory nerve endings of the skin, forming painful blisterlike eruptions or vesicles. The vesicles usually appear along a specific nerve root area called a dermatome. In some situations, reactivation of VZV may lead to dissemination of the virus to visceral and cutaneous sites (Cohen et al., 1990).

Reactivation of VZV infection in persons with HIV disease may herald the onset of other HIV-related infections. Before treatment with zidovudine became available, recurrence of VZV infection in an HIV-infected person usually meant the person would have an opportunistic infection within 1 year.

Signs and Symptoms. In primary or disseminated VZV infections, fever and chills may precede the initial eruption. The most common complaint associated with reactivated VZV infection is a burning sensation in the dermatomal area with no evidence of rash. Several days after the burning pain begins, small macular-papular vesicles begin to develop at the proximal end of the nerve. These eruptions continue to appear in a proximal-to-distal linear pattern along the dermatome. Usually the eruptions do not cross the midline of the body. Reactivation can occur in any area of the body. It is most commonly seen on the trunk. Eruptions that occur on the face frequently involve the seventh cranial nerve and may involve the eye as well.

Major complications of VZV reactivation are postherpetic neuralgia (a prolonged pain syndrome) and scarring of the infected area. Patients who are immunocompromised may have more than one episode of reactivation.

Diagnostic Evaluation. Cultures of the vesicles will be positive for VZV. However, scrapings are not usually cultured unless disseminated disease is suspected. Shingles is commonly diagnosed on the basis of the typical dermatomal appearance of the vesicles and the description of burning pain.

Treatment. Most cases of shingles are not treated and are self-limiting. Reactivation limited to one dermatome is treated with oral acyclovir, 800 mg five times a day until the lesions are dried and crusted

(Bartlett, 1992). Disseminated or facial infections generally require hospitalization. Acyclovir is given intravenously at a dosage of 30 mg/kg per day for at least 7 days.

When acyclovir is poorly effective or ineffective and cultures show acyclovir-resistant VZV, foscarnet can be used. The dosages and side effects are discussed in the section on herpes simplex viruses.

Drug Side Effects. The side effects of acyclovir are discussed in the section on herpes simplex viruses.

Sources: Kovacs & Masur, 1988; O'Dell & Zender, 1988.

Cytomegalovirus

Cytomegalovirus is a common virus that belongs to the herpesvirus family. Fifty percent of the general population of industrialized nations and 95% of the general population of nonindustrialized nations carry this virus. In industrialized nations, CMV infection is most commonly associated with lower socioeconomic status, crowded living conditions, and poor sanitation. The virus is transmitted sexually, but it can also be spread by intimate contact. It can be transmitted to the fetus in utero or to infants during birth or through breast milk. Infected children may carry the virus for long periods in the respiratory tract and urine (Flaskerud & Ungvarski, 1992).

In patients who are immunocompromised, CMV infections cause significant morbidity and mortality. Active CMV infection develops in up to 90% of patients with AIDS (Sande & Volberding, 1992). Disseminated CMV infection is an AIDS-defining condition.

Cytomegalovirus can infect the retina, lung, liver, bowel, esophagus, pancreas, blood, and central nervous system. Many clinicians attribute neuropathies, myopathies, and dementia to CMV infection. The most frequent site of infection is the eye.

Signs and Symptoms. Fever, chills, night sweats, fatigue, and malaise are the general nonspecific signs and symptoms of CMV infection. Infection of the retina can cause decreased visual acuity, floaters, and unilateral loss of vision. Examination of the eye fundi will show large, creamy, yellowish-white exudates, which are associated with hemorrhages. These must be distinguished from small, fluffy white lesions called cotton wool spots. Although common in patients with AIDS, cotton wool spots are usually asymptomatic and require no treatment. If CMV infections of the eye are left untreated, the patient will become blind.

The most common gastrointestinal infections are CMV esophagitis and colitis. The signs and symptoms are similar to those of other gastrointestinal infections. The esophagitis causes dysphagia or odynophagia. Sometimes, these are so severe the patient cannot eat or drink. Endoscopy shows ulcerous areas in the esophagus, and tests of biopsy specimens are usually positive for CMV.

Colitis caused by CMV is associated with severe, long-term diarrhea, weight loss, and anorexia. Colonoscopy shows erythematous, friable bowel, with or without ulcerative lesions. Biopsy and culture of the bowel tissue must be done to confirm the presence of CMV.

Pulmonary CMV infections are characterized by nonproductive cough, shortness of breath that gradually becomes worse, and dyspnea on exertion. When CMV is the only pathogen identified and the signs and symptoms continue to get worse, treatment with ganciclovir should be considered.

Cytomegalovirus infections of the central nervous system may cause paresthesia, sensory loss, muscle weakness, paralysis, personality changes, lethargy, and headaches.

Diagnostic Evaluation. Diagnosis of CMV retinitis is based on the clinical presentation and the retinal changes that occur in the eye. Diagnosis of CMV infection in other areas of the body is based on detection of the virus in cultures of secretions or tissue samples.

Treatment. The most important aspect of treatment is careful monitoring for visual symptoms and signs of retinal changes. Ganciclovir (DHPG, Cytovene) was the only drug available for treatment of CMV infections before foscarnet was approved at the end of 1991. Ganciclovir inhibits the growth of CMV, but it does not kill the virus. Treatment with ganciclovir stops or slows progression of CMV retinitis, causes resolution of esophagitis, and reduces the diarrhea caused by CMV colitis.

Ganciclovir is given intravenously, usually through a Hickman or Groshong central-line catheter. Initial therapy consists of an induction dosage of 5 mg/kg intravenously twice a day for 14–21 days. Because the drug does not eliminate the virus, lifelong maintenance therapy is required. The dosage for maintenance therapy is 5 mg/kg per day intravenously. When increased viral activity is evident, reinduction doses may be given and maintenance doses increased. The therapeutic effectiveness of ganciclovir for the treatment of pulmonary, colonic, and central nervous system infections has not been established, although a decrease in signs and symptoms appears to be the primary advantage of treatment.

Foscarnet is currently the drug of choice for treatment of CMV infections. Ganciclovir and foscarnet have comparable efficacy. However, unlike ganciclovir, foscarnet can be used concurrently with zidovudine, and it does not cause neutropenia.

For initial treatment, the dosage of foscarnet is 60 mg/kg every 8 hr given intravenously over 2 hr for 2–3 weeks. The dosage for maintenance therapy is 90–120 mg/kg per day given intravenously over 2 hr. Serum levels of creatinine and weight should be monitored weekly. The dosage should be adjusted if evidence of toxic effects is found.

Foscarnet irritates the vein. It must be given through a catheter in a central line. An intravenous pump is required to control the rate of infusion in order to prevent damage to the kidneys. The patient should receive an additional 1,000 ml of saline every day. If given through a peripheral vein, foscarnet should be diluted to a concentration of 12 mg/ml.

Additional information on foscarnet can be found in the other sections on viral opportunistic infections.

Drug Side Effects. The most common side effect of ganciclovir is neutropenia. Others include thrombocytopenia, eosinophilia, rash, confusion, disorientation, and phlebitis. Central venous catheter infections are a complication not related to the drug.

The major side effects of foscarnet can be found in the previous sections.

Sources: Crumpacker, 1988; Drew et al., 1988; Feinberg, 1992; Kovacs & Masur, 1988; O'Dell & Zender, 1988; Polis & Masur, 1989; Sande & Volberding, 1992.

TUMORS

As the number of HIV-positive persons has increased, the prevalence of tumors in patients with HIV disease has also increased. Several tumors are AIDS-defining conditions. The two seen most often are Kaposi's sarcoma and non-Hodgkin's lymphoma.

Kaposi's Sarcoma

Kaposi's sarcoma is the most common tumor in persons with HIV disease. It was initially described in 1872 by Moritz Kaposi, a Hungarian dermatologist. Kaposi's sarcoma is a tumor that involves the endothelial cells of blood vessels. It is unclear what causes the cells to proliferate and form a tumor. Some re-

Table 14
CATEGORIES OF KAPOSI'S SARCOMA

Category	Population Affected	Characteristics	Course
Classic	Older men (50–80 years old) of Jewish and Italian heritage	Usually confined to lower extremities; associated with venous stasis and lymphedema; male-female ratio 10–15:1	Indolent, survival 10–15 years; may be associated with other tumors
African	Young adult (25–40 years old) black men in Central Africa	Localized nodular lesions; large aggressive exophytic tumors or ones invasive to underlying bone; male-female ratio 13:1	Indolent if nodular; slowly progressive; fatal in 5–8 years
	Children (2–13 years old)	Generalized lymphadenopathy, rarely involves skin; male-female ratio 3:1	Rapidly progressive; fatal within 2–3 years
Renal transplant	Iatrogenically immunosuppressed patients; usually seen in people of Jewish or Mediterranean heritage	Involves skin only or widespread with systemic involvement; male-female ratio 2.3:1	Indolent or rapidly progressive; may regress with discontinuation of immunosuppressive therapy; 30% fatality rate
Epidemic	AIDS patients: primarily homosexual men; some Haitians, intravenous drug users, and Africans	Disseminated mucocutaneous; may involve lymph nodes, gastrointestinal and respiratory tracts	Fulminant; less than 20% survival at 2 years if opportunistic infections occur

Source: Adapted from Krigel & Friedman-Kien, 1988.

Table 15
STAGING OF KAPOSI'S SARCOMA

Stage	Clinical Features
I	Locally indolent cutaneous lesions
II	Locally aggressive cutaneous lesions
III	Mucocutaneous and lymph node involvement
IV	Visceral involvement

Subtypes

A	No systemic signs or symptoms
B	One or more systemic signs symptoms, including 10% weight loss, fever of unknown origin (body temperature greater than 100°F [38°C]) for more than 2 weeks, chills, lethargy, night sweats, anorexia, diarrhea

Source: Laubenstein, 1984.

Table 16
RECOMMENDED TREATMENT OF KAPOSI'S SARCOMA

Clinical Presentation of Lesions	Recommended Treatment
Localized	Cryotherapy, injection of antineoplastic agents, radiation therapy
Disseminated cutaneous and/or lymphadenopathic	Immunotherapy and/or single-agent chemotherapy
Aggressive, disseminated, or systemic signs and symptoms	Combination chemotherapy

Source: Adapted from Krigel, & Friedman-kein, 1988.

searchers suggest that a currently unidentified virus stimulates the cells to multiply (Volberding, 1988).

Before the advent of HIV infection, Kaposi's sarcoma was a rare tumor found primarily in older men of Italian, Eastern European, or Greek descent. Recently, the tumor has been detected in young black African males and in patients receiving immunosuppressive therapy.

Previously, Kaposi's sarcoma was divided into three categories: non-African (classic), African (endemic), and associated with transplantation. In 1981, a fourth category, AIDS-related Kaposi's sarcoma, was added. Cases of African Kaposi's sarcoma seem to be clustered near the equator. Classic Kaposi's sarcoma is seen primarily in men of Jewish ancestry or those living in the Mediterranean area (Krigel & Friedman-Kien, 1988). Table 14 (p.110) describes the four categories of Kaposi's sarcoma.

Kaposi's sarcoma is usually found on the skin. Early lesions may appear ecchymotic. Later, the lesions expand to form larger plaques or nodules. Kaposi's sarcoma frequently involves the head and neck. Appearance of a lesion within the oral cavity is often the first sign of disease. Lesions may also occur in the gastrointestinal tract, lymph nodes, liver, spleen, and respiratory tract. Patients may have a single macular or papular lesion that varies in size or multiple lesions.

The lesions in the skin rarely bleed when cut or traumatized, even though they are highly vascular. How-

Table 17
ANTINEOPLASTIC CHEMOTHERAPY FOR KAPOSI'S SARCOMA

Drug	Intravenous Dose	Schedule
Vinblastine sulfate	4 mg	Weekly
Doxorubicin hydrochloride (Adriamycin)	40 mg/m^2	Day 1
Vinblastine sulfate	150 mg/m^2	Day 1
Bleomycin sulfate	15 units/m^2	Day 1, 15 (cycle repeats every 21 days)
Etoposide (VP-16)	150 mg/m^2	Day 1,2,3 (cycle repeats every 28 days)
Doxorubicin hydrochloride (Adriamycin)	40 mg/m^2	Day 1
Vinblastine sulfate	6 mg/m^2	Day 1 (cycle repeats every 21 days)
Doxorubicin hydrochloride (Adriamycin)	20 mg/m^2	Day 1
Vinblastine sulfate	4 mg/m^2	Day 1
Bleomycin sulfate	15 units/m^2	Day 1, 15
Dactinomycin (Actinomycin D)	1 mg/m^2	Day 8
Vincristine sulfate	1.4 mg/m^2	Day 8
Dacarbazine (DTIC - Dom)	375 mg/m^2	Day 8 (cycle repeats every 28 days)

Source: Adapted from Moran, 1988.

ever, in later stages of gastrointestinal Kaposi's sarcoma, slow bleeding may result from erosion of the tumor. Although Kaposi's sarcoma is usually not a cause of death, it contributes to morbidity. Lesions may grow to the point where they restrict movement and become painful. Also, the tumors often cause lymphatic obstruction, leading to severe edema.

Staging systems have been proposed to account for the variations in Kaposi's sarcoma and to monitor progression. The systems are based on clinical features. Each system has its limitations. Volberding (1988) has suggested that prognosis in patients with AIDS should be related to overall clinical status, levels of P24 antigen and $_2$-microglobulin, blood cell counts, and results of biochemical tests. Prognosis is worse when the patients also have opportunistic infections. Table 15 (p.111) describes the system most commonly used to stage Kaposi's sarcoma.

Signs and Symptoms. The lesions of Kaposi's sarcoma are brown, purple, or reddish-purple. They may be nodular, flat, round, or oval. New lesions have a yellow-green halo. The lesions are usually painless unless they extend over bone prominences or affect areas with minimal skin surface.

Diagnostic Evaluation. Presumptive diagnosis of Kaposi's sarcoma is based on the appearance of the lesions. Definitive diagnosis of skin lesions is based on the results of biopsy.

Treatment. Currently, no effective therapies for treatment or prevention of Kaposi's sarcoma are available. Palliative therapy is designed to decrease the progression of lesions or modify their appearance. Treatments are local or systemic. Recommendations for treatment are listed in Table 16.

Local treatments are designed to modify the appearance of the lesions or the effects of the lesions on organ systems. Cryotherapy decreases the size or intense color of the lesions on the exposed surfaces of the body. Liquid nitrogen is the most common form of cryotherapy.

Vinblastine sulfate and tumor necrosis factor injected into lesions have decreased their size. Dinitrochlorobenzene (DNCB) has also been applied topically to small lesions. Local therapy for larger lesions has been ineffective.

Radiation therapy is probably the most common form of local therapy. Low doses are effective for small lesions, especially those on the skin and mucous membranes. Radiation also has been used to reduce edema associated with lymphatic invasion. Its effectiveness depends on the extent of lymphatic involvement and the amount of surrounding tissue necrosis that occurs.

Systemic treatment consists of chemotherapy. Treatment with chemotherapeutic agents may make the underlying immunodeficiency associated with AIDS worse. Also, it is difficult to achieve complete remission of the tumors. Chemotherapy with a single agent

---

Table 18
ANN ARBOR STAGING SYSTEM FOR NON-HODGKIN'S LYMPHOMA

Stage	Degree of Involvement
I	Involvement of a single lymph node region or a single extralymphatic organ or site
II	Involvement of two or more lymph node regions, or localized involvement of one or more extralymphatic organs or sites on the same side of the diaphragm
III	Involvement of lymph node regions on both sides of the diaphragm, which may also be accompanied by localized involvement of an extralymphatic organ or site, by involvement of the spleen, or both
IV	Diffuse, disseminated involvement of one or more extralymphatic organs or tissue, with or without associated lymph node enlargement

Source: Adapted from DeVita & Hellman, 1982.

---

is used for lesions that are cutaneous and progressing slowly. Rapidly progressing lesions are treated with multiple agents, with limited success. Table 17 (p.112) lists the chemotherapeutic agents and dosages used.

Treatment with alpha and beta interferons and interleukin-2, separately or in conjunction with other chemotherapeutic agents (such as zidovudine), is currently being studied. Results to date have been mixed.

Therapy and Drug Side Effects. The most significant side effect of radiation therapy to the head, face, and mouth is mucositis. The most common side effects of chemotherapy are pancytopenia, hair loss, fatigue, nausea, vomiting, diarrhea, and weakness (Volberding, 1988.)

Lymphomas

Lymphomas are tumors of the immune system. Four types are seen persons with HIV disease: non-Hodgkin's lymphoma, B-cell lymphoma, Burkitt's lymphoma, and primary lymphoma of the central nervous system.

Non-Hodgkin's Lymphoma

Non-Hodgkin's lymphoma may be the first clinical evidence of HIV infection, or it may appear after the occurrence of opportunistic infections. It is the most common lymphoma in people with HIV infection. The cause is unknown.

Signs and Symptoms. Non-Hodgkin's lymphoma appears as a painless enlargement of a lymph node, usually on one side of the body. The signs and symptoms are nonspecific. They may include fever, night sweats, or weight loss greater than 10% of the patient's total body weight (Flaskerud & Ungvarski, 1992). The tumor gradually enlarges and spreads to the adjacent lymphatics and other organs. The liver, spleen, gastrointestinal tract, respiratory tract, and central nervous system may be involved. Other signs and symptoms are related to the organ or organs involved. These include increased intracranial pressure, nausea, vomiting, elevated levels of liver enzymes, cough, shortness of breath, fever, chills, and night sweats.

Diagnostic Evaluation. Diagnosis is based on histologic examination of biopsy specimens of the tumor. Staging of the tumor is based on the involvement of organ systems. The most common system is the Ann Arbor Staging System (DeVita & Hellman, 1982). Table 18 (p.113) lists the stages in this system.

Treatment. Treatment is based on the stage of the disease. The following chemotherapeutic agents are generally used in combination: cyclophosphamide (Cytoxin), vincristine sulfate, methotrexate, etoposide (VP-16), cytarabine (ara-C), bleomycin sulfate, and corticosteroids. In some cases, surgery is used for localized lesions. Radiation therapy may also be used in conjunction with chemotherapy or surgery.

B-Cell Lymphoma

Although relatively uncommon, B-cell lymphomas in HIV-positive persons have been reported. They are seen more often in homosexual men than in any other group infected with HIV.

The tumors involve the lymphatic system and other organs. New evidence suggests that this lymphoma may be caused by EBV or be related to infection with this virus. Signs and symptoms, diagnosis, and treatment are similar to those for non-Hodgkin's lymphoma.

Burkitt's Lymphoma

Burkitt's lymphoma is the second most common lymphoma in persons with HIV disease. It is associated with EBV. The tumors are found in the lymph nodes and major organ systems. Occasionally, multiple organ sites are involved simultaneously. Signs and symptoms are related to the organ or organs involved. Diagnosis is based on histologic examination of affected tissue. Treatment is similar to that of non-Hodgkin's lymphoma (Volberding, 1988.)

Primary Lymphoma of the Central Nervous System

Primary lymphoma of the central nervous system in persons with acquired and genetic immunodeficiencies has long been recognized. The most common signs and symptoms are headache, nausea, vomiting, focal defects, seizures, and altered mental status.

Diagnosis is based primarily on findings on CT scans of the head. If possible, biopsy of the tumor for tissue classification should be done. CT scans show

Table 19
CLINICAL SIGNS AND SYMPTOMS OF AIDS DEMENTIA COMPLEX

Early Manifestations	Late Manifestations

Cognitive
 	
   Impaired concentration
   Mental slowing
   Memory loss
 	
Motor
 	
   Leg weakness
   Unsteady gait
   Tremor
   Loss of coordination, impaired handwriting
 	
Behavioral
 	
   Agitation, confusion, hallucinations
   Apathy, withdrawal, "depression"
 	
Mental Status
 	
   Psychomotor slowing
   Organic psychosis
   Impaired serial 7s or reversals
 	
Neurologic
 	
   Release reflexes (snout, glabellar, grasp)
   Gait ataxia (impaired tandem gait, rapid turns)
   Impaired rapid movements (limbs, eyes)
   Tremor (postural)
   Leg weakness
   Hyperreflexia
	Mental Status
	
	   Global dementia
	   Unawareness of illness, disinhibition
	   Confusion, disorientation
	   Organic psychosis
	   Psychomotor slowing (verbal responses delayed, near or absolute mutism, vacant stare)
	
	Neurologic
	
	   Ataxia
	   Weakness (legs more than arms)
	   Pyramidal tract signs (spasticity, hyperreflexia, extensor plantar responses)
	   Myoclonus
	   Urinary and fecal incontinence

For related text, see page 116.

Source: Adapted from Brew, Rosenblum, & Price, 1988.

Table 20
STAGING SYSTEM FOR AIDS DEMENTIA COMPLEX

Stage	Degree of Dementia	Signs and Symptoms
0	Normal	Normal mental and motor function.
1	Mild	Able to perform all but the more demanding activities of daily living. Evidence of motor and intellectual impairment on neurologic testing. Can walk without assistance.
2	Moderate	Able to perform activities of self-care but cannot work. Able to walk but may require a single prop.
3	Severe	Major intellectual impairment. Cannot follow news or personal events, sustain complex conversations. Output is slowed. Motor function is clumsy, and assistance is required.
4	End Stage	Nearly vegetative. Intellectual and social comprehension and output are at a rudimentary level. May be mute, incontinent, and unable to walk or assist self.

Sources: Aronow, Brew, & Price, 1988; Brew, Rosenblum, & Price, 1988; Carr, Newlin, & Gee, 1988.

ring-enhancing lesions. The lesions must be distinguished from those caused by toxoplasmosis. In general, the lesions caused by toxoplasmosis are smaller than those caused by lymphoma. Treatment is radiation therapy and management of signs and symptoms. Chemotherapy with the same drugs used for treatment of other lymphomas is also being tried. Success has varied. Currently, no other effective treatment is available.

AIDS DEMENTIA COMPLEX

The precise cause of AIDS dementia complex (ADC) is unknown. Also known as subacute encephalitis and AIDS encephalopathy, ADC is the most common neurologic syndrome in persons with HIV disease. Signs and symptoms include decreased memory, inability to concentrate, apathy, and psychomotor retardation. These manifestations are usually recognized on the basis of the cognitive, behavioral, and motor triad and are slowly progressive.

AIDS dementia complex may be the first manifestation of HIV infection. More often, however, it is preceded by one or more opportunistic infections. Since 1987, ADC has been an AIDS-defining condition.

The possible pathogenic mechanisms of ADC are numerous. Infected macrophages and multinucleated cells are probably responsible for the spread of HIV to the brain. Viral antigens have also been detected in microglial and astrocytic tumor cell lines (Aronow, Brew, & Price, 1988)

Signs and Symptoms. The signs and symptoms of ADC have a subtle onset. They are also difficult to differentiate from the signs and symptoms of other illnesses, such as Alzheimer's and Parkinson's diseases and depression. Table 19 (p.115) presents the manifestations of the early and late stages of ADC. Aronow et al. (1988) found it helpful to use a staging system for clinical management and research purposes (see Table 20, p.116).

Diagnostic Evaluation. Diagnosis of ADC requires a thorough history, confirmation of HIV infection, and evidence of neurologic signs and symptoms. A spinal tap and a CT scan of the head should be done. Often CT scans show cerebral atrophy that does not correspond with the stated age of the patient. This tends to be a later sign of ADC. Cerebrospinal fluid will have elevated level of protein with no other abnormalities. The results of these tests will also rule out other potential causes for the changes in mental status.

Neuropsychiatric testing should be completed to support clinical findings. These tests show characteristic abnormalities in complex sequencing, impairment of fine and rapid motor movement, and slowed verbal fluency.

Treatment. No effective treatment of ADC is available. Because HIV infection of the central nervous system is the most likely cause of ADC, treatment of the infection is the recommended course of action. Treatment with zidovudine has had the most effect. It may prevent or slow down progression of ADC. In some patients taking zidovudine, confusion and cognitive and motor deficits have disappeared (Brew, Rosenblum, and Price, 1988; Price, Brew, & Roke, 1992). They reappeared when treatment with the drug was stopped.

Because of the lack of adequate therapies, management of the various signs and symptoms and maintenance of a safe environment are the best treatments.

EXAM QUESTIONS

Chapter 7

Questions 48 - 64

48. When an organism that ordinarily does not cause disease in a person with a healthy immune system causes an infection in someone whose immune system is weakened, the term used to describe the infection is:

    a. Pathogenic
    b. Opportunistic
    c. Communicable
    d. Nosocomial

49. Which protozoan is the major cause of focal intracerebral lesions in patients with AIDS?

    a. *Pneumocystis carinii*
    b. *Isospora belli*
    c. *Toxoplasma gondii*
    d. *Cryptosporidium* species

50. Which of the following organisms commonly cause diarrhea in persons with HIV infection?

    a. *Salmonella* and *Shigella*
    b. *Candida* and *Cryptococcus*
    c. Herpes simplex virus and cytomegalovirus
    d. *Cryptosporidium* and *Pneumocystis*

51. What is the medication of choice for treatment of infection caused by *Cryptococcus neoformans*?

    a. Amphotericin B
    b. Ketoconazole
    c. Zidovudine
    d. Dideoxycytidine

52. Which protozoan invades tissues, causing cell death and a severe inflammatory process?

    a. *Toxoplasma gondii*
    b. *Isospora belli*
    c. *Pneumocystis carinii*
    d. *Giardia lamblia*

53. The eye is the most common site of infection for which virus in persons with HIV disease?

    a. Herpes simplex virus
    b. Varicella-zoster virus
    c. Epstein-Barr virus
    d. Cytomegalovirus

54. Which drugs are licensed by the Food and Drug Administration for treatment of cytomegalovirus infections?

    a. Acyclovir and ganciclovir
    b. Foscarnet and zidovudine
    c. Ganciclovir and foscarnet
    d. Zidovudine and acyclovir

55. The most common lymphoma in patients with HIV disease is:

    a. B-cell lymphoma
    b. Primary lymphoma of the central nervous system
    c. Burkitt's lymphoma
    d. Non-Hodgkin's lymphoma

56. Shingles is caused by what organism?

    a. Herpes simplex virus
    b. Varicella-zoster virus
    c. Cytomegalovirus
    d. Epstein-Barr virus

57. Rash, nausea, vomiting, and diarrhea are side effects of which two drugs used to treat toxoplasmosis?

    a. Pyrimethamine and nicotinic acid
    b. Pyrimethamine and sulfadiazine
    c. Sulfadiazine and clindamycin
    d. Clindamycin and nicotinic acid

58. Which of the following drugs has shown some effect in the treatment of AIDS dementia complex?

    a. Zidovudine
    b. Haloperidol
    c. Acyclovir
    d. Ganciclovir

59. Which of the following statements about *Mycobacterium tuberculosis* (MTB) and *Mycobacterium avium-intracellulare* (MAI) is correct?

    a. MTB infection is restricted to the lungs.
    b. MTB rarely causes infection in patients with HIV disease.
    c. MAI is the most frequent opportunistic infection in patients with AIDS.
    d. MAI infections are often not detected until autopsy.

60. The most common side effect of acyclovir is elevated levels of:

    a. Blood urea nitrogen and creatinine
    b. Liver enzymes and albumin
    c. Cholesterol and triglycerides
    d. Sodium and potassium

61. Early manifestations of AIDS dementia complex include:

    a. Disinhibition and release reflexes
    b. Global dementia and pyramidal tract signs
    c. Impaired concentration and memory loss
    d. Disorientation and psychomotor slowing

62. What disorder in patients with AIDS is characterized by psychomotor slowing, organic psychosis, global dementia, and myoclonus?

    a. AIDS dementia complex
    b. Toxoplasmic encephalitis
    c. HIV psychosis
    d. Cytomegalovirus infection of the central nervous system

63. Which of the following organs are sites of infection for cytomegalovirus?

    a. Retina, lung, liver, bowel, blood, central nervous system
    b. Retina, lung, liver, bowel, skin
    c. Lung, blood, skin, mouth
    d. Retina, central nervous system, bladder, liver

64. What is the most common side effect of flucytosine?

    a. Nausea
    b. Diarrhea
    c. Rash
    d. Headache

CHAPTER 8

NURSING CARE

CHAPTER OBJECTIVE

After studying this chapter, the reader will be able to describe nursing care problems of persons infected with HIV, specify appropriate nursing diagnoses and interventions, and develop a plan of care for these problems.

LEARNING OBJECTIVES

After studying this chapter, the reader should be able to

1. Define the nurse's role in caring for persons with HIV disease.

2. Specify the appropriate level of nursing care activities for patients with HIV disease who are hospitalized.

3. Specify the process used to determine nursing care activities.

4. Indicate the steps in the nursing process.

5. Explain the term *outcome criteria*.

6. Explain why evaluating the plan of care is important.

7. Specify two nursing diagnoses for anorexia, nausea, and vomiting.

8. Select a correct nursing intervention for anxiety.

9. Choose two outcome criteria appropriate for depression.

10. Indicate a nursing diagnosis for diarrhea.

11. List three appropriate outcome criteria for impaired mobility.

12. Select the appropriate nursing diagnosis for fever.

13. Specify the correct problem(s) for a nursing diagnosis statement of alteration in physical regulation related to infection with HIV or opportunistic organisms.

14. Specify the correct area of the nursing process for the following statement: Add individualized nursing interventions specific to the patient.

15. Select the correct nursing diagnosis for pain.

16. Choose the correct problem for the outcome criteria statement of alteration in self-concept.

INTRODUCTION

The nurse's role is to support maximal well-being, regardless of the patient's life circumstances such as illness, pain, poverty, ignorance, or death. Nursing care throughout the ages has been directed toward management or resolution of signs and symptoms. Outcome criteria define the expected status or the changes to be achieved by a specified time, for example, before the patient is discharged from the hospital. Many of these criteria are defined by all-or-none terms such as *absence, free from,* or *able to.*

Nursing care of patients with HIV disease involves support of their maximal well-being, management of signs and symptoms, and health maintenance rather than cure or resolution. Outcome criteria continue to define the expected status or changes to be achieved. For patients with HIV disease, however, criteria that include the absolutes of all or none are inappropriate, and they should be modified to reflect the compromised immune status of the patient. Outcomes related to management or lessening of the problem by the patient or the patient's significant other are more appropriate.

Nursing interventions are similar to those used with other medical-surgical diagnoses. Planning for the nursing care of a patient with HIV disease requires considering the entire spectrum of the illness. Flaskerud & Ungvarski (1992) have described a three-tiered system to determine appropriate nursing activities for care of patients with HIV disease:

Primary level	Nursing activities directed toward health appraisal
Secondary level	Nursing activities directed toward health protection
Tertiary level	Nursing activities directed toward minimizing residual disabilities related to progression of HIV infection or AIDS and maximizing the quality of life

NURSING PROCESS

Planning nursing care for persons infected with HIV uses the nursing process and nursing diagnosis. The nursing process involves assessment (history, physical, diagnostic tests), nursing diagnosis, interventions, and evaluation. This process is continuous, as shown in Figure 14.

Nursing diagnosis is a specific way to define a type of problem detected by nurses. It provides a method for describing a person's health status in clear and concise ways that enhance communication and planning (Carpenito, 1983). A nursing diagnosis has three components: (1) a label or title that describes the actual or potential state of the person's health, (2) etiology or contributing factors, and (3) defining characteristics. The label uses qualifying terms such as *alteration, impaired, deficit,* or *ineffective* to reflect changes in health status.

Once the actual or potential problems are detected, nursing activities are planned. Nursing interventions

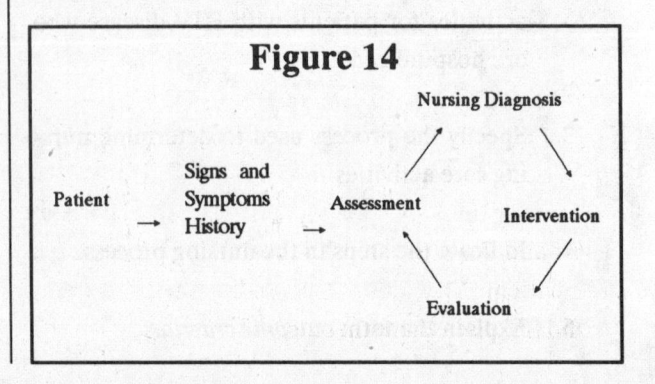

Figure 14

Patient → Signs and Symptoms History → Assessment → Nursing Diagnosis → Intervention → Evaluation

CHAPTER 8 — NURSING CARE

are the activities nurses do to prevent, reduce, minimize, or eliminate the defined problem (nursing diagnosis). Intervention has four components: (1) establishing priorities of care, (2) determining expected outcomes, (3) setting nursing goals, and (4) initiating the plan through nursing orders. Outcome criteria focus on the patient's goals or the changes expected in the patient after nursing care is received. Nursing goals are the actions a nurse takes to prevent, minimize, or alleviate the altered health state. Outcome criteria must be measurable and are qualified by verbs such as *accepts, knows, states, performs, administers, has a decrease or increase in,* and *identifies* (Carpenito, 1983).

Achieving expected outcomes for patients depends on two factors. The first is an appropriate and accurate health appraisal and physical examination. The second is determination of the appropriate related-to or secondary-to statements of the nursing diagnosis. For patients with HIV disease, establishment of realistic outcome criteria will result in more appropriate nursing interventions. Outcome criteria and nursing interventions give direction for discharge planning.

The final aspect of the nursing process is evaluation. Evaluation is continuous and should enable the nurse to modify outcome criteria and interventions according to changes in the nursing diagnosis or the patient's condition. Evaluation also enables the nurse to determine if outcome criteria and nursing interventions have been completed.

PLANNING NURSING CARE

Planning nursing care is based on the patient's signs and symptoms and the results of evaluation of the patient. The most common findings in patients with HIV disease are the following:

Weight loss	Pain
Skin problems	Depression
Fever	Sweats
Chills	Diarrhea
Nausea	Vomiting
Oral lesions	Fatigue
Weakness	Wasting
Cough	Shortness of breath
Anorexia	Edema
Anxiety	Fear
Knowledge deficits	

The most frequently used nursing diagnoses applicable to these findings are

Alterations in nutrition
    Less than body requirements
    Impaired swallowing
    Loss of appetite

Alterations in physical regulation
    Potential infection
    Body temperature

Alterations in circulation
    Fluid volume deficits

Alterations in elimination
    Bowel: diarrhea or constipation
    Bladder: control of or retention

Alterations in oxygenation
    Impaired gas exchange
    Ineffective airway clearance
    Ineffective breathing pattern
    Airway obstruction

Alterations in physical integrity
    Potential for injury
    Impairment of skin integrity
    Alterations in oral mucous membranes

Alterations in socialization

Social isolation
Alterations in role
Alterations in work

Alterations in sexual patterns

Alterations in coping
Ineffective individual
Ineffective family, friends, lovers

Alterations in activity
Impaired physical mobility

Alterations in recreation
Diversional activity deficits

Alterations in self-care
Self-care deficits

Alterations in self-concept
Disturbance in self-concept

Sensory-perceptual alterations
Visual, kinesthetics

Alterations in meaningfulness
Hopelessness
Powerlessness

Alterations in knowledge and thought process
Knowledge deficits
Confusion
Memory loss

Alterations in comfort
Acute or chronic

Alterations in emotional integrity
Anxiety
Fear
Grieving

These findings and nursing diagnoses are used to develop the outcome criteria and nursing interventions described in the following pages. These care plans are examples. They do not include every potential problem, nursing diagnosis, outcome criteria, or nursing intervention. They should be considered examples rather than established standards of care.

CHAPTER 8 — NURSING CARE

CARE PLANS FOR PATIENTS WITH HIV DISEASE

Problem: Anorexia, nausea, vomiting

Nursing Diagnosis	Outcome Criteria	Nursing Interventions
Alteration in nutrition related to anorexia related to nausea or vomiting	Participates in activities to enhance nutritional status	Keep a weekly record of weight
Alteration in tissue perfusion related to vomiting related to inadequate nutrition related to knowledge deficit	Carries out regimen to take in adequate fluids and nutrition	Keep a record of fluid and calorie intake
	States ways to increase fluids and nutrition	Discuss eating habits
	States appropriate use of antiemetics	Discuss changes in eating habits to increase fluid and calorie intake
	States what to do if unable to maintain nutritional status	Discuss resources available to help with shopping, meal preparation, meal delivery, feeding
	States appropriate resources for support	Discuss use of antiemetics
	States ways to control coughing	Modify medication regimen to reduce nausea and vomiting associated with medications
	Improved skin turgor and electrolytes	Instruct patient on techniques to control cough
		Add individualized nursing interventions specific to patient

125

Problem: Anxiety

Nursing Diagnosis	Outcome Criteria	Nursing Interventions
Alterations in emotional integrity related to prognosis related to change in socioeconomic status related to coping patterns related to treatments and procedures	Identifies factors that increase or decrease anxiety Verbalizes reasons for anxiety Takes steps necessary to decrease anxiety Uses coping strategies appropriately and effectively States appropriate resources for support Verbalizes knowledge and understanding of treatments and procedures	Establish a therapeutic relationship with patient Provide opportunity for patient to verbalize feelings, concerns, anxieties Help patient identify and use coping strategies Explain all treatments and procedures simply and concisely Assess and document patient's readiness to learn, coping mechanisms, and skills Inform patient about and provide a list of support services Add individualized nursing interventions specific to patient

CHAPTER 8 —
NURSING CARE

Problem: Cough

Nursing Diagnosis	Outcome Criteria	Nursing Interventions
Alterations in respiratory function related to infection	Promotes optimal respiratory function	Explain how to do controlled deep breathing and controlled coughing and help patient do these procedures
Ineffective airway clearance related to sputum production related to chronic, unrelieved cough related to obstruction	Minimizes discomfort associated with cough	Demonstrate and reinforce breathing patterns and techniques
Impaired gas exchange related to secretions related to bronchospasm	Demonstrates effective coughing and increases air exchange	Explain use of medications to control cough
	Verbalizes understanding of the use of medications and fluids to decrease cough	Encourage hydration: 2–3 L of fluid per day
		Add individualized nursing interventions specific to patient

Problem: Depression

Nursing Diagnosis	Outcome Criteria	Nursing Interventions
Alteration in emotional integrity related to illness Ineffective individual coping related to depression	Verbalizes feelings about emotional state Identifies coping patterns Identifies personal strengths and receives support through the nursing relationship Makes decisions and follows through with appropriate actions Increases coping ability and effectiveness	Establish a therapeutic relationship with the patient Provide atmosphere of acceptance Provide opportunities for expression of feelings, fears, anxieties about self and others Add individualized nursing interventions specific to patient

CHAPTER 8 —
NURSING CARE

Problem: Diarrhea

Nursing Diagnosis	Outcome Criteria	Nursing Interventions

Alteration in bowel elimination related to opportunistic infection related to medications related to diet intolerance	Describes contributing factors when known
	Identifies methods of reducing contributing factors
	Explains rationale for interventions
	Experiences less diarrhea
	Describes methods to prevent dehydration, loss of electrolytes, breakdown of skin
		Determine causative factors
		Reduce or eliminate contributing factors:
		  diet
		  medications
		  causative organism
		Increase fluid intake and low-residue diet
		Encourage patient to eat frequent small meals
		Encourage use of antidiarrheal agents
		Explain rationale for medications
		Add individualized nursing interventions specific to patient

Problem: Edema

Nursing Diagnosis	Outcome Criteria	Nursing Interventions
Fluid volume excess related to nutritional deficits related to low serum albumin related to obstruction	Reduction of swelling in extremities Relates causative factors and methods of preventing or minimizing edema	Assess for swelling Discuss causative factors and possible interventions Encourage increased intake of protein and fat Encourage patient to eat frequent small meals Encourage elevation of extremity to reduce swelling Add individualized nursing interventions specific to patient

CHAPTER 8 —
NURSING CARE

Problem: Fatigue

Nursing Diagnosis	Outcome Criteria	Nursing Interventions
Alteration in activity related to AIDS related to insufficient oxygen transport secondary to pneumonia related to depression	Identifies factors that affect activity tolerance Identifies methods to increase activity tolerance and promote independence in activities of daily living Performs activities safely without increased dyspnea or fatigue	Discuss activity intolerance Determine a schedule that allows adequate rest by coordinating all activity, treatments, and activities of daily living Assess oxygen status and seek oxygen replacement Teach safety precautions to prevent falls Teach proper use of walking aids Add individualized nursing interventions specific to patient

Problem: Fear

Nursing Diagnosis	Outcome Criteria	Nursing Interventions
Alteration in emotional integrity Fear related to uncertainty of illness related to treatments and procedures related to death and dying related to hospitalization related to reaction of others to diagnosis related to isolation and stigmatization	Differentiates between real and imagined fears Recognizes effective and ineffective coping patterns Verbalizes fears to improve psychologic and physiologic comfort Gains knowledge related to the fear, how fear may be modified, and available resources for support	Assess for evidence of fear Assess for contributing factors: unfamiliar environment change in life-style biological changes threat to self-esteem Use self (nurse) as therapeutic mechanism to decrease fear Provide opportunity to express feelings, concerns, questions Provide opportunity to verbalize etiologic factors and how to cope with them Develop teaching plan to decrease fears related to hospital, procedures, medications, equipment Add individualized nursing interventions specific to patient

CHAPTER 8 —
NURSING CARE

Problem: Fever

Nursing Diagnosis	Outcome Criteria	Nursing Interventions

Alteration in temperature regulation
Hyperthermia related to HIV or opportunistic infection
Fluid volume deficit related to abnormal fluid loss
	Controls or minimizes fever
	Experiences minimal associated discomfort
	Replaces fluid loss and maintains electrolyte balance
	Demonstrates ability to take and record body temperature correctly
	States appropriate interventions for an elevated body temperature:
	  antipyretics
	  cooling measures
	  notification of care provider
		Monitor vital signs, especially body temperature
		Assess for and document associated signs:
		  chills
		  rigors
		  tachycardia
		  sweats
		  tachypnea
		  loss of skin turgor
		Administer antipyretics as ordered
		Evaluate need for cooling measures such as tepid sponges, cool shower, cooling mattress
		Eliminate excessive clothing and bed linen
		Encourage fluid intake or increase amount of fluids
		Provide dry clothes and bed linen
		Assess patient's ability to take and record body temperature
		Instruct patient on when to
		  take temperature
		  take acetaminophen, aspirin, or other antipyretics
		  inform care provider
		  use other measures to decrease body temperature
		Add individualized nursing interventions specific to patient

Problem: Impaired mobility

Nursing Diagnosis	Outcome Criteria	Nursing Interventions
Alteration in activity related to motor dysfunction because of neurologic involvement related to wasting and debilitation	Absence of skin breakdown Achieves optimal level of activity that promotes physical mobility Engages in activities without injury Remains as independent as possible	Assess patient's activity level Establish a schedule that supports patient's need for activity, rest, and sleep Assist with activities of daily living as needed Exercise muscles and joints as tolerated Encourage ambulation and other activities as tolerated Provide necessary equipment (e.g., walker, wheelchair) to enable ambulation and activity Encourage change in body position every 2 hr to prevent skin breakdown Instruct patient on ways to increase mobility and exercise and prevent skin breakdown Add individualized nursing interventions specific to patient

CHAPTER 8 —
NURSING CARE

Problem: Infection, infection control

Nursing Diagnosis	Outcome Criteria	Nursing Interventions
Potential for infection related to immunosuppression Potential for transmission of HIV related to knowledge deficit	Shows no or minimal signs and symptoms related to infection States procedures to follow to prevent, detect, and treat infections Prevention of nosocomial infections States and demonstrates infection control procedures	Assess and document signs and symptoms related to infection Monitor skin, mouth, rectum, and intravenous sites for evidence of infection Monitor vital signs on a regular basis Instruct patient on monitoring for signs and symptoms of infection Instruct patient on procedures to follow when evidence of infection is present Alert physician about signs and symptoms of infection Administer appropriate medication to treat infections Follow infection control procedures Instruct patient on infection control procedures Add individualized nursing interventions specific to patient

CHAPTER 8 — NURSING APPROACHES TO HIV/AIDS CARE

Problem: Isolation

Nursing Diagnosis	Outcome Criteria	Nursing Interventions
Potential for social isolation related to hospitalization rejection because of homophobia prejudice fear social stigma inadequate social support systems changes in life-style interpersonal skills	Able to acknowledge current level of socialization Discusses ways to improve socialization Patient's feelings of social isolation are minimized States resources available to increase support	Use self (nurse) as therapeutic agent Discuss expected health care outcomes and previous socialization patterns Confront behaviors detrimental to socialization Explore alternatives to increase socialization Discuss resources and opportunities to socialize Add individualized nursing interventions specific to patient

CHAPTER 8 — NURSING CARE

Problem: Nausea and vomiting

Nursing Diagnosis	Outcome Criteria	Nursing Interventions

Alteration in circulation related to potential deficiency in fluid volume	Describes causative factors and identifies ways to minimize them
	Identifies fluid and nutrition loss and ways to decrease the loss
	Relief of signs and symptoms of dehydration
	Control of cough (see care plan for additional outcomes)
		Assess for signs and symptoms of volume depletion:
		  decrease in skin turgor
		  dry mucous membranes
		  weight loss
		  orthostatic hypotension
		  dizziness, blackouts
		Monitor intake and output
		Administer antiemetics as prescribed
		Encourage intake of frequent small amounts of fluids, ice chips, or food
		Provide good mouth care before patient eats
		Encourage patient to eat small frequent meals (up to six to eight per day)
		Allow patient to select food items or preferences
		Administer cough medications as prescribed
		Add individualized nursing interventions specific to patient

Alterations in nutrition related to nausea or vomiting related to coughing		

Problem: Oral lesions, dysphagia, odynophagia

Nursing Diagnosis	Outcome Criteria	Nursing Interventions
Alteration in mucous membranes related to Kaposi's sarcoma related to fungal, herpetic, or CMV lesions Alteration in nutrition related to oral or esophageal lesions	Alleviates or minimizes discomfort from lesions in mucous membranes Maintains optimal integrity of mucous membranes Maintains fluid and electrolyte balance Increases nutritional intake	Assess mucous membranes and fluid and nutrition status each shift Develop plan to maintain or improve condition of mucous membranes Provide good oral hygiene Apply moisturizer to lips as needed Administer medications as prescribed Instruct patient on importance of good oral hygiene and taking medications as prescribed Provide adequate fluids and nutrition Add individualized nursing interventions specific to patient

CHAPTER 8 —
NURSING CARE

Problem: Pain

Nursing Diagnosis	Outcome Criteria	Nursing Interventions

Alteration in comfort
    related to peripheral neuropathies
    related to pressure on nerve endings because of lesions or tumors
    related to immobility
    related to involvement of central nervous system
    related to infections
    related to medications
	Obtains maximum pain relief from pain control measures
	States choices of pain control measures (e.g., medication, music, meditation)
	States medications, dosing schedule, actions, and side effects
		Assess for character and intensity of pain and note sudden changes in degree of pain (use pain scale of 1–10)
		Eliminate pain stimulus:
		    unnecessary movement
		    muscular tension
		    prolonged periods in one position
		Assess need for pain medications and monitor effects of pain medications
		Determine pain medication schedule for control of pain
		Administer pain medications on a regular basis for chronic pain
		Provide alternative measures for pain relief
		Facilitate patient's self-control over pain:
		    allow choices in care and methods of pain control
		    provide information about procedures and treatments
		    encourage use of alternative measures
		Instruct patient and family about pain medication, alternative therapies, and diversional activities
		Add individualized nursing interventions specific to patient

CHAPTER 8 — NURSING APPROACHES TO HIV/AIDS CARE

Problem: Shortness of breath

Nursing Diagnosis	Outcome Criteria	Nursing Interventions
Impaired gas exchange related to hypoxemia because of opportunistic infections pneumonia pleural effusion radiation therapy pneumothorax medications depression of central nervous system related to pain related to ineffective airway clearance related to thick secretions related to ineffective cough related to ineffective breathing pattern related to severe cough or dyspnea associated with Kaposi's sarcoma pneumonia tuberculosis bacterial, fungal, or viral infections diagnostic procedures	Improved gas exchange Adequate level of oxygenation, based on disease state Experiences relief from or minimal dyspnea, inadequate oxygen, and weakness Demonstrates effective coughing Carries out activities of daily living with minimal exertion, fatigue, and respiratory distress Minimizes anxiety and discomfort associated with respiratory changes Demonstrates appropriate use of equipment	Assess respiratory status for evidence of distress, impaired gas exchange, and hypoxia Encourage coughing to maintain patent airway Use suctioning as necessary to maintain patent airway Monitor use and effectiveness of oxygen, mechanical ventilation, humidification, chest tubes, and medications Help patient find positions for comfortable breathing Help with activities of daily living as needed Organize nursing care to permit periods of rest Maintain hydration Provide medications that decrease anxiety related to respiratory distress Administer pain medications as needed Instruct patient on ways to increase activity without increasing shortness of breath Provide instructions on how to use equipment Add individualized nursing interventions specific to patient

CHAPTER 8 — NURSING CARE

Problem: Skin problems

Nursing Diagnosis	Outcome Criteria	Nursing Interventions

Alterations in physical integrity
Impaired skin integrity (actual or potential)
  related to HIV
  related to Kaposi's sarcoma
  related to effects of immobility
  related to poor nutritional status
  related to prolonged skin contact with body secretions
  related to allergic reactions
  related to edema
  related to skin disorders
	Maintains skin integrity or minimizes skin breakdown, rashes
	Healing of skin, wound, to optimal status
	Maintains nutrition and fluid intake
	Verbalizes and demonstrate treatments
	Demonstrates proper care of wound or skin
	Verbalizes ways to avoid skin breakdown
		Assess skin surfaces every shift for redness, breakdown, and lesions and document findings
		Keep skin dry and clean; provide skin care as needed
		Assist with bath and massage skin with lotion
		Clean and pat dry rectal and perineal areas after each bowel movement
		Follow institution's decubitus staging and treatment
		Provide appropriate bed, mattress pads, air mattress, or other equipment
		Encourage patient to change body position every 1–2 hr
		Establish and post routine for change in body position for bed-bound patient
		Provide clean clothing and bed linen as needed
		Maintain adequate nutrition and hydration
		Instruct patient on ways to improve skin integrity, prevent skin breakdown, and care for wounds and lesions
		Add individualized nursing interventions specific to patient

Problem: Wasting, weight loss

Nursing Diagnosis	Outcome Criteria	Nursing Interventions
Alteration in nutrition related to anorexia related to nausea or vomiting related to inability to obtain food	Identifies factors that contribute to weight loss	Assess for signs and symptoms of malnutrition or weight loss
Alteration in bowel elimination related to opportunistic infection related to medications related to diet intolerance	Eliminates, minimizes, or controls nausea, vomiting, mouth problems, odynophagia, dysphagia, diarrhea, ability to obtain food	Help patient identify reasons for weight loss
Alteration in mucous membranes related to Kaposi's sarcoma related to fungal, herpetic, or CMV lesions related to odynophagia or dysphagia	Verbalizes and/or demonstrates ways to eliminate, minimize, or control causes of wasting or weight loss	Monitor weight, intake and output of food and fluids
Alteration in self-concept	Verbalizes feelings about change in physical image	Provide medications to control or minimize anorexia, nausea, vomiting, and diarrhea
		Encourage good oral hygiene
		Provide medications to eliminate or minimize odynophagia, dysphagia, mouth lesions or soreness
		Encourage intake of foods high in calories, including food supplements
		Instruct patient on ways to increase caloric intake
		Provide for appropriate community assistance with shopping, meal preparation or provision (e.g., Meals on Wheels)
		Instruct on medications, actions, and side effects to prevent nausea, vomiting, diarrhea, mouth lesions, odynophagia, dysphagia
		Provide atmosphere for patient to verbalize feelings relating to body image and emotional changes
		Add individualized nursing interventions specific to patient

CONCLUSION

Nursing has the opportunity to meet the challenge of the decade. HIV infection and AIDS have no cure, and patients with HIV disease need intensive care and services. No other profession can support maximal well-being regardless of the patient's life circumstances. It is currently up to nursing to provide support that enhances the life of the patient and helps maintain health and well-being.

The next chapter discusses discharge planning and management of home and ambulatory care.

Sources: California Nurses Association, 1987; Carpenito, 1983; Flaskerud & Ungvarski, 1992; MacIntyre, Tueller, & Wishon, 1988; Wesorick, 1990.

EXAM QUESTIONS

Chapter 8

Questions 65 - 74

65. Having a patient with HIV infection verbalize feelings and identify personal strengths would be an appropriate outcome criterion for which sign or symptom?

    a. Anger
    b. Isolation
    c. Depression
    d. Panic

66. What level of nursing care activities is appropriate for a patient with HIV disease who is hospitalized?

    a. Primary
    b. Secondary
    c. Tertiary
    d. Intermediate

67. Support of a patient's maximal well-being regardless of the patient's life circumstances such as illness, pain, poverty, ignorance, or death is the definition of which of the following?

    a. Nursing care
    b. Nurse's role
    c. Nursing process
    d. Nursing intervention

68. Helping a patient with HIV disease identify and use appropriate coping strategies is a nursing intervention that can be used for which common sign or symptom?

    a. Depression
    b. Anxiety
    c. Wasting
    d. Pain

69. Alteration in bowel elimination is a nursing diagnosis for what common HIV-related problem?

    a. Anorexia
    b. Diarrhea
    c. Edema
    d. Nausea and vomiting

70. Absence of skin breakdown and remaining as independent as possible are possible outcome criteria for which AIDS-related health care problem?

    a. Wasting and weight loss
    b. Skin problems
    c. Weakness
    d. Impaired mobility

CHAPTER 8 —
NURSING CARE

71. Which of the following is used by nurses to determine the plan of care for patients with HIV infection?

    a. Nursing process
    b. Nursing care plan
    c. Patient care plan
    d. Primary care nursing

72. Alteration in nutrition and alteration in tissue perfusion are nursing diagnoses for which AIDS-related health problem?

    a. Wasting, weight loss
    b. Oral lesions, dysphagia, odynophagia
    c. Anorexia, nausea, and vomiting
    d. Edema

73. Which of the following is a sign or symptom seen in HIV infection and AIDS that would have alteration in physical regulation related to hyperthermia as a nursing diagnosis?

    a. Fever
    b. Weakness
    c. Fatigue
    d. Diarrhea

74. Alteration in comfort is a nursing diagnosis for which of the following health problems in a patient with HIV disease?

    a. Fever
    b. Pain
    c. Shortness of breath
    d. Wasting

CHAPTER 9

DISCHARGE PLANNING, HOME AND AMBULATORY CARE

CHAPTER OBJECTIVE

After studying this chapter, the reader will be able to identify the home care needs of patients with AIDS, specify a discharge plan to meet those needs after hospitalization, and recognize problems in ambulatory care and specify appropriate nursing interventions.

LEARNING OBJECTIVES

After studying this chapter, the reader should be able to

1. Specify the three health care systems coordinated by the case manager.

2. Describe the role of the case manager.

3. Indicate when discharge planning should begin.

4. Select the components of discharge planning.

5. Choose the benefits of discharge planning.

6. Indicate the barriers to discharge planning.

7. Describe the Karnofsky Scale.

8. Specify the advantages of home health care.

9. Select the services available in the home care setting.

10. Specify the stages of illness that determine the level of home health care.

11. Recognize the role of the home health nurse.

12. Explain why the home health nurse assesses social support systems and psychologic status.

13. Specify the most common signs and symptoms detected during home health care of patients with HIV disease.

14. Indicate the services that should be available in the ambulatory care setting.

15. Describe the services provided by nurse screening clinics.

16. Suggest topics that should be included in patient education.

INTRODUCTION

Nursing care of patients with HIV disease presents unique opportunities in any setting. The ongoing health care problems that frequently result in hospitalization begin in the patient's own environment. Problems normally taken care of by hospitalization are never fully solved for those who have HIV disease. Outcome criteria for problems diagnosed by nurses must be modified to meet discharge goals. Innovative approaches are required to meet the needs of the patient and the patient's life partners (spouse or lover), family, and friends. Many communities cannot or do not provide services that will enable the patient to remain in the home, and often coordination between the hospital, home, and outpatient care is lacking.

NURSING CASE MANAGEMENT

Care of patients with HIV disease requires a management system that includes hospital, ambulatory, and home care. Coordination between these three systems requires effective communication, timely assessment, flexibility, and the collaboration of care providers. One method of coordinating these systems is nursing case management.

Nurse case managers work with health care providers and the patient's significant others to coordinate care and services in the hospital, home, and ambulatory care settings. They assist both the patient and the health care providers. The case management system preserves human dignity, provides for informed choice, and seeks to ensure safe care (Nyamathi & Hedderman, 1989). The case manager also facilitates the patient's movement through the health care system and provides continuity of care and a holistic approach to the needs of the patient and the patient's significant others.

Case managers assess the patient's physical, mental, financial, and social status in all three settings. Interventions are based on the ongoing assessments, interventions, and evaluations. The care plan is determined by the patient's needs and priorities and the results of the nurse's assessment. The plan is then discussed with those involved in the patient's care, including the physician when appropriate.

Case management is the key to coordinating health care outside the hospital. It links and integrates home, hospital, clinic, and community resources. Case management enables nurses to apply the full scope of professional practice and to participate in critical decisions about the efficiency of health care.

DISCHARGE PLANNING

Discharge planning begins with admission to the hospital. Plans are based on assessment of the patient's problems; determination of functional level; determination of equipment, service, and educational needs; available resources (financial and personal); and social support. Meetings are held with the patient, members of the patient's support sys-

CHAPTER 9 —
DISCHARGE PLANNING, HOME AND AMBULATORY CARE

tems, physicians, social workers, and nurses. The purpose is to determine the current level of care and to estimate the level of care that will be needed after discharge from the hospital. Time frames for therapies and education should be discussed in these meetings, and use of community services and follow-up care should be determined and arranged before the patient leaves the hospital.

The first step in discharge planning is the nursing assessment done at admission. This assessment should include the following: evaluation of signs and symptoms, physical status, functional level, support systems (those reported by the patient and those reported by the members of the support system), financial status, living environment, and outpatient follow-up. Each area assessed provides an indication of the patient's ability to function on discharge and helps determine a realistic discharge plan.

An important part of ongoing discharge plans is determining the functional level of the patient. This information gives a good indication of the patient's ability to provide self-care. Determination of functional level should be part of the nurse's daily assessment. Several instruments are currently used by hospitals throughout United States. The most common one in the ambulatory care setting (which may also be used in the hospital setting) is the Karnofsky Scale (Carter, Glatstein, & Livingston, 1982; Table 21, p.150).

The Karnofsky Scale combines signs and symptoms with activity level to determine functional level. This scale, or a modification of it designed to fit a particular client's needs, can be used to determine the needs of the patient at home after discharge. These needs include education, equipment, and care. The case description given later in this section shows how to use the Karnofsky Scale to determine discharge plans and the care and services that will be needed during ambulatory care.

Discharge planning is an important part of the nursing care plan in the hospital. Use of diagnosis-related groups (DRGs) to control length of hospitalization and hospital costs has resulted in early discharge. Because of early discharge, many patients and the patients' significant others may not be prepared to return home and provide care. With early discharge planning, patients can remain in the home environment longer. Lack of an appropriate discharge plan may result in frequent visits to emergency departments or admissions to the hospital or both.

In many hospitals, discharge planning is the responsibility of the discharge planner. Some facilities use case managers from the community to help with discharge planning for special groups of patients. Nurses need to determine who is providing this service within their hospital and be prepared to plan the discharge for all patients assigned to their care. Discharge planning is not the responsibility of just one person; all nurses are responsible.

Incorporating discharge planning in the hospital care is difficult when most patients are acutely ill. Nurses and other staff members normally are caught up in providing acute care, with little thought given to the patient's needs on discharge. The patient's degree of illness, however, is not a satisfactory reason for little or no discharge planning.

Discharge planning has four benefits: (1) hospital and community services save money; (2) hospital beds are more readily available; (3) relapses, needless hospital stays, and unnecessary emergency visits are decreased; and (4) staff members, patients, families, and others are actively involved in the care and planning. Involvement in planning enables everyone to take part in making decisions. This leads to satisfaction, responsibility, and accountability for patients and staff members.

Discharge planning has several barriers. Two of the most important are lack of communication between

Table 21
THE KARNOFSKY SCALE: CRITERIA OF PERFORMANCE STATUS

Status	% of Normal	Criteria
Able to carry on normal activity, no special care is needed	100	Normal, no complaints, no evidence of disease
	90	Able to carry on normal activity, minor signs or symptoms of disease
	80	Normal activity with effort, some signs or symptoms of disease
Unable to work, able to live at home and care for most personal needs, a variable amount of assistance needed	70	Cares for self, unable to carry on normal activity or to do active work
	60	Requires occasional care for most needs
	50	Requires considerable assistance and frequent medical care
Unable to care for self, requires equivalent of institutional or hospital care, disease may be progressing rapidly	40	Disabled, requires special care and assistance
	30	Severely disabled, hospitalization is indicated although death not imminent
	20	Very sick, hospitalization necessary, active supportive treatment necessary
	10	Moribund; fatal processes progressing rapidly
	0	Dead

Source: Adapted from Carter, Glatstein, & Livingston, 1982.

care providers and lack of knowledge of community resources. Communication between nurses, physicians, and patients must be ongoing. Nurses need to continually assess the functional level of the patient. The physician should be included in discussions early in the patient's hospital stay about the planned discharge date and potential equipment and medication needs. Failure to communicate important information is the major reason for inadequate or inappropriate discharge plans. For patients with HIV disease, failure to communicate important information about the home environment and social support systems may result in the patient's being discharged to inadequate housing or care or readmitted to the hospital within a short time.

Information about community resources is also important. Knowledge of financial systems can help patients obtain some type of income if they cannot work. Financial resources include social security, state disability funds, company disability or pension plans, veterans' benefits, and private insurance benefits. Community services such as medical care providers, home health care agencies, public health nursing services, and support groups are valuable for assisting and maintaining the patient within the home environment. Many patients with HIV disease are receiving intravenous therapy or injectable medications at home, which require the assistance of nursing services. Other community services such as physical therapy, day care, or transportation may be required by patients who are weak or unable to stay alone during the day (Stanhope, Sheahan, & Kent, 1984).

Other barriers to effective discharge planning are failure to determine home care needs and waiting until the day of discharge to arrange for services. Discharge plans made in haste may not adequately address all the home care needs. Persons who make up the patient's support systems may need to rearrange work schedules so they can provide needed care or simply be available to the patient. Some patients may have lost housing before they were hospitalized. Finding a new place to live may take days to weeks. Little financial support and housing are available for most persons who are HIV-positive. For patients who are terminally ill, securing sufficient support in the home environment is difficult even in the best of circumstances. Obtaining a bed in a long-term care facility; additional equipment, such as a bedside commode; and equipment for oxygen and intravenous therapy may take several days.

Example of Discharge Planning

The following case study demonstrates the importance of discharge planning. It also illustrates the importance of early planning and of including the patient's significant others and community services.

J. L. is a 32-year-old black man who uses injectable drugs. He has been admitted to the hospital for the first time with anemia and fever. He lives on the streets and receives money from the county welfare program. His nursing history indicates that he has used intravenous heroin, crystal, and methamphetamines. He last used drugs 3 days before admission. He has lost 40 lb (18 kg) over the past 2 months. He has been having fevers (exact body temperature unknown because he does not own a thermometer), chills, and sweats for several weeks. He has several brothers and sisters who live in the same town but who do not want to associate with him. He was married for several years and has two children. He does not know the current location of his wife or children.

On admission, physical findings are as follows: body temperature, 103°F (39°C); pulse, 104 beats per minute; respirations, 28/min; and blood pressure, 100/60 mm Hg. Hemoglobin and hematocrit are 8.6 g/dl and 23.5, respectively. The patient is weak, cannot undress himself without assistance, and becomes fatigued with minimal exertion. According to the Karnofsky Scale (Table 21), J. L.'s functional level on admission is 30%.

Over the next several days, J. L. receives multiple blood transfusions, and tests are done to determine the cause of his fever and anemia. He continues to become easily fatigued and cannot perform all his activities of daily living. His fever persists (body temperature, 39°C). His functional level continues to be 30–40%.

On day 10 in the hospital, he is informed that he is seropositive for HIV and has an acid-fast bacillus growing in his blood. The bacillus is thought to be *M. avium-intracellulare*. He is started on medication: rifampin, ciprofloxacin, and clofazamine by mouth and amikacin by intramuscular injection. The presence of MAI in the blood is an AIDS-defining condition. The social worker applies for state disability, social security, and veterans disability for J. L. and begins discussing future housing with him. The nurse makes a referral to a community home health care agency.

On day 15, J. L.'s body temperature decreases to 100°F (38°C), and his energy level increases despite nausea and occasional vomiting caused by the medications. He is able to do most of his activities of daily living, but he continues to become easily fatigued. His functional level is now 50–60%. The medical staff decides J. L. will be ready for discharge in 4–5 days. His projected functional level on discharge is 60–70%.

The Karnofsky Scale, the initial and ongoing social and physical assessment, and input from J. L. are used to form the following discharge plans:

Referral to a case management system
Placement in an AIDS residential care facility
Community nursing visits daily for amikacin injections, physical assessment, and emotional support
Assistance with medications
In-home support services to assist with homemaking chores and activities of daily living
Medical follow-up in a community-based clinic
A wheelchair to assist with ambulation
Education relating to
   AIDS diagnosis
   Reduction of risk factors
   Prevention of transmission of HIV
   Infection control in the home
   Diet and fluids
   Monitoring of body temperature and other physical changes that may indicate increasing or new health problems
   Medications

Over the next 7 months, J. L.'s functional level increases to 80%, and his need for assistance in the residential care facility decreases. Injections of amikacin have been stopped. Treatment with zidovudine has been started, along with Septra DS for PCP prophylaxis. J. L. is seen every 2–4 weeks in the outpatient clinic at the hospital. He continues to become easily fatigued, occasionally has a fever, and is unable to work. He now receives social security disability and supplemental social security income.

During the eighth month after discharge, J. L.'s fever recurs (body temperature up to 104°F [40°C]). He has chills, sweats, fatigue, shortness of breath, and cough. He is readmitted to the hospital with anemia. Pneumocystis pneumonia is diagnosed. His functional level is 20%. After treatment, his functional level increases to 40%, and plans are made for him to return to the residential care facility. Plans for discharge at this time include the following:

Continued case management
Continued medical follow-up
Increase in homemaker services
Special equipment (e.g., hospital bed, bedside commode, walker)
Attendant care to assist with bathing and general comfort care
Increase in visits by community nurse to monitor care given by the attendant and to determine additional service needs

HOME HEALTH CARE

Health care within the home or community setting can control costs and provide humane care to patients with AIDS. Home health care reduces the length of hospital stays and the frequency and number of hospitalizations (Little, Long, & Kehoe, 1990).

Home health care offers a wide range of services for patients with HIV disease. These include skilled nursing care; social services; home health aides; and physical, occupational, speech, intravenous, and respiratory therapy.

Providing care in the hospital is one thing. Providing care in the home is another. Equipment, supplies, assistance, and support from physicians are always readily available in the hospital, and nursing practice is guided by standard procedures, protocols, and physician's orders. In the home care setting, physician's orders also guide nursing services, medi-

CHAPTER 9 —
DISCHARGE PLANNING, HOME AND AMBULATORY CARE

cations, and treatment. However, makeshift protocols and standards of care that require ingenuity and imagination often are standard operating procedures in this setting. Education and clear communication must guide those who provide care in the home.

The focus of home health care depends on the patient's stage of illness. One patient's care may focus on maintaining and regaining independence. Another's may focus on assistance in managing chronic signs and symptoms. For patients who are terminally ill, the focus is palliative care to provide support until death occurs.

To determine the focus of home health care, nurses use the nursing process to detect problems and plan interventions. This process is the same as that used to identify problems in the hospital setting (see Chapter 8). The home environment should be carefully assessed to detect risk factors that might prevent the patient from remaining at home. Areas to be considered are safety, infection control, physical and emotional status, support systems, medication management, inadequate education, and financial resources.

Risk factors are assessed by obtaining a thorough history and doing a physical examination during the initial visit to the home. Table 22 (p.154–155) is an example of a home health assessment form.

Developing a home care plan begins with identifying the patient's perception of the illness. Comprehensive evaluation of physical and emotional concerns and the environment (living arrangements) enables the nurse to develop a plan that includes realistic goals for optimal comfort. The patient's description of signs and symptoms should alert the nurse to the patient's most pressing problems. These must be addressed first before other issues can be managed.

Effective management of signs and symptoms depends on the physical and emotional status of the patient and the patient's personal support systems. The most common (and most debilitating) signs and symptoms in the home care environment are pain, anorexia, nausea, vomiting, fever, chills, sweats, diarrhea, fatigue, fear, anxiety, and depression. Depression, oral candidiasis or HSV infection, nausea, vomiting, anorexia, and diarrhea create nutritional problems that can lead to weight loss. Soft foods, drinks made in a blender, and canned nutritional supplements may help increase caloric intake. Frequent small meals or more constant intake of food and beverages (snacking) are better than three meals a day. Having foods available that require no preparation can prevent fatigue and encourage eating. Also, the addition of foods with a sharp taste, such as lemons, limes, raspberries, cranberries, or vinegar, may encourage intake of bland foods.

Chronic fatigue, especially in the later stages of illness, is a barrier to self-care, dietary intake, and maintenance of environment. Homemaker services that shop for and prepare meals and do the housekeeping will enable the patient to stay in the home environment and decrease fatigue. Table 23 (p.157–158) contains suggestions for managing other common signs and symptoms.

Home health nurses, home health aides, and homemaker and in-home support services provide much of the actual physical care required by patients with HIV disease. Patients who are maintaining and regaining functional status may require physical therapy. Respiratory therapy is commonly used during the chronic and palliative stages of the illness. Nutritional therapy is required by all patients who receive health care at home. This includes oral supplements, intravenous therapies, and tube feeding.

Home health nurses are actively involved in assessing the environment for possible safety hazards. Stairs and rugs can be hazardous for patients who are weak, easily fatigued, and unsteady. Lack of sufficient heat, air circulation, lighting, running water, and toilet facilities poses infection-control and physi-

Table 22
SAMPLE ASSESSMENT FORM FOR HOME HEALTH CARE OF AIDS PATIENTS

Name:
Address:
Phone:
Emergency Contact: Code Status:
Physician/Practitioner:

Level of Function

Opportunistic Infections/Malignant Tumors

1. Disease stage: maintaining/regaining, chronic, palliative
2. Functional status: ____ (Karnofsky Scale)
3. Independence in activities of daily living
4. Level of activity: works, moderate, minimal, housebound, bedbound

1. Candidiasis (oral, esophageal, perineal)
2. *Pneumocystis carinii* pneumonia
3. Toxoplasmosis
4. Cryptococcal infections
5. Herpes simplex (oral, perianal, genital, rectal)
6. Herpes-zoster (localized, disseminated)
7. Cytomegalovirus (eye, esophagus, colon, lung, other organs)
8. *Mycobacterium avium intracellulare* (MAI)
9. *Mycobacterium tuberculosis*
10. *Cryptosporidium*
11. Histoplasmosis
12. Coccidioidomycosis
13. Progressive multifocal leukoencephalopathy (PML)
14. Non-Hodgkin's lymphoma
15. Burkitt's lymphoma

5. Requires assistance with
   a. All activities of daily living
   b. Bowel and bladder care
   c. Feeding
   d. Bathing
   e. Getting in and out of bed or chair
   f. Ambulation
   g. Meal preparation
   h. Shopping
   i. Transportation
   j. House cleaning and maintenance

Medications and Treatments

Social Assessment

1. Financial resources
2. Living situation
3. Social support systems
   Lover   Friends
   Family   Groups
4. Community resources
5. Case manager
6. Healthcare provider(s)
7. Home health services
8. Transportation

Sign and Symptom Review

General
   Temperature, pulse, blood pressure
   Overall appearance

Table 22 (continued)

Skin
- Intact
- Rash
- Lesions
- Edema
- Breakdown (location and size)

Pulmonary
- Shortness of breath: sitting, walking, walking distance, tires easily
- Cough: productive, nonproductive
- Oxygen: type and rate
- Physical examination: respiratory rate, breath sounds

Gastrointestinal
- Appetite/hydration/intake: solids, fluids, supplement, intravenous
- Nausea/vomiting: frequency, timing, amount
- Bowels: continent/incontinent
- Diarrhea: frequency, timing, amount
- Constipation: bowel program, rectal pain
- Physical examination: mouth, bowel sounds, tenderness, perianal or rectal lesions

Genitourinary
- Continent/incontinent
- Catheter: type
- Physical examination: rash, lesions, skin breakdown

Case Manager:

Durable Power of Attorney:

Other Directives:

Neurological
- Headache with/without nausea/vomiting
- Visual changes
- Focal weakness or loss of function
- Seizures
- Pain
- Gait changes
- Physical examination: eyes, pupils, reflexes, strength, vibratory/position, coordination

Mental
- Alert and oriented
- Disoriented/confused
- Memory lapses or forgetfulness
- Drowsy
- Difficult to arouse
- Unarousable/comatose

Assessment

Interventions

cal problems. Weakness and fatigue can also affect the patient's ability to provide self-care.

Besides providing direct nursing services, the home health nurse is instrumental in educating the patient and the patient's significant others, family members, roommates, and friends. Education on how to prevent transmission of HIV and on infection control is the nurse's responsibility. The nurse must also give instruction on medications and their side effects and on the goals of treatment plans.

The nurse should also educate the patient's family, friends, roommates, and significant others about the availability of community resources. Knowledge of available resources will help patients use services to the best advantage. Many of these services provide additional support that enables patients to remain in the home environment for longer periods or until death.

The home health care nurse often is the person best able to assess the patient's social support systems. Some patients who have AIDS have many persons available to provide care and supportive functions. Others have minimal or no support systems. For many reasons, patients with AIDS are frequently separated from their biological families. This separation may have occurred because of rejection, anger, or prejudice about the patient's sexual orientation or life-style. Others have sought separation so their lifestyle would be unknown to their families. Separation from traditional families has resulted in the creation of nontraditional families consisting of significant others, adopted parents, and friends.

All those involved in the life of a patient with AIDS may become part of the patient's support system. Accurate assessment of this system is crucial to maintaining the patient in the home environment. It is not uncommon for a patient to claim that many persons are available to provide care and services in the home. However, when the home health nurse arrives, the actual number of caregivers turns out to be none, one, or two. Many potential members of a support system may be able to provide assistance only occasionally. Accurate assessment, adequate support systems, and service resources may enable the very ill or terminally ill patient to remain at home.

Psychosocial issues must be assessed at each home visit. These issues affect both the patient and the persons who make up the patient's support system. Many of the psychologic issues revolve around the complexity of the disease process, curative vs. palliative therapy, and bereavement issues (Lieberman, 1988).

Multiple recurrent opportunistic infections create a roller coaster ride for the patient and the members of the patient's support system. The signs and symptoms of the infection get worse and then improve along with signs and symptoms of physical and/or mental deterioration. Aggressive treatment cannot stop the overall destruction of the immune system, and eventually the patient dies. No one knows which episode or worsening of signs and symptoms and infections may be a warning of imminent death. This situation increases anxiety and fear. Eventually, the patient and the members of the patients's support system must make decisions about further treatment and care.

Because of the ever-present hope of a cure, patients with AIDS are ambivalent about therapy programs. Many seek palliative care (measures that provide comfort only) while seeking experimental curative treatments for HIV infection. The ultimate decision on when to stop treatments for cure is up to the patient (or a designated decision maker if the patient is incompetent). Ongoing discussions that present all the facts help the patient or others make timely and appropriate decisions. The home health nurse who maintains open communication and permits ongoing dialogue about curative and palliative therapy allows the patient to make choices about care and treatment and have control over some aspects of life.

CHAPTER 9 —
DISCHARGE PLANNING, HOME AND AMBULATORY CARE

Table 23
MANAGEMENT OF SIGNS AND SYMPTOMS IN AIDS

Sign or Symptom	Medication	Nursing Intervention
Anorexia	Megestrol acetate (Megace) 20–40 mg orally three times a day	Encourage intake of favorite foods, small meals, strongly flavored foods.
Anxiety	Lorazepam (Ativan) 0.5–2.0 mg orally three times a day	Discuss fears, concerns.
	Diazepam (Valium) 2–10 mg orally three times a day	Permit ventilation of anger, fears.
	Morphine sulfate 2–10 mg orally, subcutaneously, or intravenously every 4–6 hours	
Cough	Cough medications with dextromethorphan hydrobromide or codeine 1–2 teaspoons orally every 4 hours	Instruct on cough control techniques.
	Codeine 30 mg orally every 4–6 hours	
	Elixir of terpin hydrate with codeine 1–2 teaspoons every 4–6 hours	
Depression	Tricyclic antidepressants	Encourage to ventilate anger, discuss fears and concerns.
	Amitriptyline (Elavil) 25–150 mg orally at bedtime	
Diarrhea	Kaopectatin (Kaopectate) 1–2 tablespoons after each stool	Force fluids, especially those high in calories and electrolytes, such as Gatorade, Pedialyte.
	Psyllium hydrophilic mucoloid (Metamucil) 1 tablespoon in glass of water	
	Diphenoxylate hydrochloride and atropine sulfate (Lomotil) 1–2 tablets after each stool or every 4–6 hours	Increase flour products such as pasta, bread, crackers.
	Loperamide (Imodium) 2 mg, 1–2 tablets after each stool or every 4–6 hours	Decrease or eliminate milk products.
	Codeine 30 mg orally every 4–6 hours	
	Paregoric 5 ml orally four times a day	
	Tincture of opium 0.6 ml orally four times a day up to 6 ml/day in divided doses	
	Dicyclomine hydrochloride (Bentyl, Bentylol) 10–20 mg orally three or four times a day	
Fever	Acetylsalicylic acid (aspirin) 650 mg orally with food or rectally every 4–6 hours as needed or around the clock	Force fluids.
		Reduce clothing and bedding.
	Acetaminophen (Tylenol) 650–1,000 mg orally with food or rectally every 4–6 hours as needed or around the clock	Encourage cool baths or shower.
	Ibuprofen (Motrin, Advil, Nuprin) 400–800 mg orally with food every 4–6 hours as needed or around the clock	
	Naproxen (Naprosyn) 250–375 mg with food every 6–8 hours as needed or around the clock	

Table 23 *(Continued)*

Signs or Symptom	Medication	Nursing Intervention
Nausea or Vomiting	Prochlorperazine (Compazine) 10–25 mg orally or rectally every 4–6 hours as needed or around the clock Lorazepam (Ativan) 0.5–2.0 mg orally every 6–8 hours as needed or around the clock Metaclopramide (Reglan) 0.2–2.0 mg/kg orally or intravenously every 8 hours Trimethobenzamide (Tigan) 200–250 mg orally or rectally every 6 hours as needed or around the clock Thiethylperazine (Torecan) 10 mg orally or rectally every 8 hours as needed Dronabinol (Marinol; synthetic form of an antiemetic compound found in marijuana) 2.5–10.0 mg orally every 4–6 hours	Encourage intake of frequent small amounts of fluids: broth, juices, tea, electrolyte-replacing (mix electrolyte-replacing fluids in strongly flavored juices to mask taste). Provide ice chips, frozen juice chips, frozen electrolyte fluids. Give fluids, foods, and medications 30–60 minutes after the antiemetics.
Pain	Acetaminophen (Tylenol) 650–1,000 mg orally or rectally every 4–6 hours as needed or around the clock Acetylsalicylic acid 650 mg orally or rectally every 4–6 hours as needed or around the clock Ibuprofen (Advil, Motrin, Nuprin) 400–800 mg orally every 6–8 hours as needed or around the clock Naproxen (Naprosyn) 250–375 mg orally every 6–8 hours as needed or around the clock Codeine 30–60 mg orally every 4–6 hours as needed Oxycodone (Percodan) 5 mg orally every 4–6 hours as needed or around the clock Hydromorphone (Dilaudid) 2–12 mg orally, subcutaneously, or intramuscularly every 2–4 hours as needed or around the clock Meperidine hydrochloride (Demerol) 25-100 mg orally or intramuscularly every 4–8 hours as needed Morphine sulfate 2–100 mg orally, subcutaneously, or intravenously every 2–12 hours as needed or around the clock Methadone (Dolophine) 5–25 mg orally or intramuscularly every 4–12 hours as needed or around the clock Amitriptyline (Elavil) 25–150 mg orally at bedtime or every 12 hours Haloperidol (Haldol) 0.5–5.0 mg orally or intramuscularly four times a day or every 6 hours as needed or around the clock Fentanyl transdermal (Duragesic) 25–100 mg/hr patches	Provide medication on a regular basis to provide better pain control. Start with lower dose and work up. Control cause of pain (e.g., herpes, candidiasis, inflammation). Use heat or cold; can alternate. Elevate swollen limbs. Increase range of motion. Reposition bed patients frequently. Change subcutaneous sites every 3–4 days. Rotate intramuscular injection sites. Add patches, which last 72 hours, to increase dose; rotate sites. Use other oral narcotics also if break-through pain occurs.

Bereavement issues for patients who are terminally ill vary. The most common ones are fear of pain and death caused by a debilitating disease, loss of independence and control, and disfigurement and changes in body image and sexuality. Patients with AIDS also fear avoidance, rejection, and isolation by friends and family members as death nears.

Many patients with AIDS deal not only with their own fears and losses but also with the losses of lovers, friends, and family members who died of AIDS. Depression and feelings of helplessness and hopelessness are common.

Home health nurses must be prepared for all the ups and downs these patients present. Being alert for and addressing the issues of death, loss, and isolation or rejection will foster appropriate coping and acceptance by the patient and the members of the patient's support system. Nurses should also be prepared for the patient's denial early in the stages of chronic and terminal illness. In some situations, denial is an appropriate coping mechanism that makes it possible to deal with intolerable situations and maintain hope.

AMBULATORY CARE

Patients with HIV disease may receive outpatient care in a clinic or an office (further references to clinic denote both clinic and office). This care is episodic and depends on the physical and emotional status of the patient. Several health care providers, including physicians, nurse practitioners, and physician assistants, are frequently involved in the clinical management of these patients. In this setting, the nurse is the ideal person to provide initial and continuing assessment of the patients' physical, emotional, financial, and social status. In settings with multiple practitioners, the nurse provides the continuity.

The ambulatory care setting is frequently the first health care contact for persons infected with HIV. Many clinics treat the entire spectrum of HIV disease. Others may limit their HIV practice to patients who are asymptomatic or to patients who are symptomatic or who have a diagnosis of AIDS. Clinics should provide screening, referral, education, diagnosis, treatment, and follow-up care.

Ambulatory care provides both primary and secondary levels of nursing care (see chapter 8). Primary nursing care (health maintenance) focuses on an organized appraisal of the patient's health status. The secondary level of care focuses on nursing activities that prevent development of infections in the immunocompromised patient (Ungvarski, 1989).

Nurse screening clinics for HIV infection have been established in many areas. These clinics use both primary- and secondary-level nursing activities. The clinics provide (1) screening services for the asymptomatic and the symptomatic, (2) access to a medical system knowledgeable about HIV infection, (3) preliminary tests to facilitate assessment by a physician, and (4) a systematic approach to the nursing assessment of patients. The nurse's activities are guided by protocols or algorithms (Carr, Newlin, & Gee, 1988).

Persons at risk for HIV infection are encouraged to be tested for HIV before signs and symptoms develop. Those who are infected can start treatment with zidovudine early and can learn about HIV disease. Initial and subsequent visits to the clinic should include assessment of risk factors; educational needs; and physical, mental, social, and financial status. Persons with HIV infection who are asymptomatic may require only periodic visits. These persons usually have CD4 counts higher than 500 cells/mm^3.

Patients who have HIV infection and those who have AIDS may require more frequent assessments and interventions in the ambulatory care setting as more knowledge about treatment of infections and tumors becomes available. Knowledge about treatments and about changes in the patient's physical and emotional status will enable the nurse to make appropriate interventions and referrals. Most of the information on infections and tumors, treatment of infections and tumors, and nursing care is presented in chapters 6–8. Knowledge of the patient's current physical and emotional status also enables the nurse to make appropriate referrals to community services and agencies.

Nurses in any setting play a major role in preventing the spread of HIV. All patients and their significant others, regardless of the stage of infection, should receive education about the disease process, the plan of care, and ways to prevent transmission of HIV. Knowledge of risk factors allows the nurse to intervene with appropriate education. Table 24 (p.161–162) lists areas that should be discussed with patients and the patients' significant others.

The patient's ability to manage the necessary medications may also be a problem. Compliance is difficult, especially when taking medications reminds patients that they have a terminal illness. Using "pill minder" boxes (small boxes with alarms) or establishing a routine that reminds the patient when to take the medications is helpful. Also, once-a-day medications do not have to be taken all at the same time as long as they are taken every day. Splitting the medications up decreases the amount taken at any one time and may decrease the amount of gastrointestinal upset.

Assessment for disability also occurs most often in the outpatient setting. Determining the patient's ability to perform normal work activities may be difficult, especially if an inability is related to emotional problems rather than to physical status or a diagnosis of AIDS. Often the nurse is in the best position to know a patient's ability to perform work or other daily activities. This information is obtained through casual conversations with the patient and the patient's significant others. If depression or dementia is suspected, then psychiatric evaluation and psychologic testing will be important for an accurate assessment of emotional status.

Applications for disability, general relief, or pensions can be a paperwork maze for many patients. Knowing about disability forms and requirements for state and social security disability benefits will help patients complete their applications. The U.S. Social Security Administration and the Department of Veterans Affairs require documentation of an opportunistic infection or tumor before a request for disability can be completed. Obtaining and sending this documentation along with the application will help the agencies process claims faster.

CONCLUSION

Ambulatory care includes home health care and outpatient care in the office or clinic. Management of HIV-infected individuals within these settings requires a different type of nursing skill. Subtle changes in physical and mental status may be detected because most patients are seen many times during their illness. Assessment techniques and interventions require the nurse to be innovative and creative. Communication and observation skills and logical reasoning are needed to recognize problems and draw important conclusions.

Use of a case management system that works in the inpatient, outpatient, and home care settings is the best way to maximize patients' satisfaction, continuity of care, and coordination of services. Case management by a nurse or team within these settings is unique to the nursing profession. The ultimate result of such a system is timely and appropriate interventions and efficient and effective care.

The next chapter discusses the psychosocial implications of HIV infection and AIDS.

CHAPTER 9 —
DISCHARGE PLANNING, HOME AND AMBULATORY CARE

Table 24
EDUCATIONAL TOPICS FOR PATIENT WITH AIDS

Topic	Details to Cover
HIV Disease	**Definition** **Causes** **Stages of illness** **Differences between asymptomatic HIV disease, symptomatic HIV disease and AIDS**

Risk Factors	**Sexual**
	   Multiple partners
	   Infected partner
	   Partner who uses injectable drugs
	   Homosexual or bisexual partner
	
	Use of injectable drugs
	   Users
	   Partner of a user
	
	Infants of a seropositive mother

Transmission	**Sexual** **Use of injectable drugs** **Untested blood products** **Infected mother to child**

Prevention	**Sexual Abstinence**
	Safe sex
	   Use latex condoms (preferably with nonoxynol-9)
	   Avoid exchange of body fluids during sexual activity
	   Avoid multiple partners
	   Avoid unknown partners
	   Avoid partners who use drugs
	
	Do not use injectable drugs or any street drugs, including alcohol
	
	Use of injectable drugs
	   Do not use
	   Do not share works
	   If works shared, clean them with diluted bleach
	   Use latex condoms and nonoxynol-9 during sex
	
	Pregnancy
	   Avoid if seropositive
	
	Do not share toothbrushes or razors

Table 24 (continued)

Prevention (*continued*)	Clean toilets, bathrooms, and spills of blood or other body fluids with bleach (one part bleach to nine parts water), hot water, and detergent, or other household disinfectants
	Dispose of needles and razors in rigid containers, paper products in leak-proof plastic bags
	Wash dishes, bedding, and clothes in hot water with detergent
	Wear gloves to clean up blood and other body fluids
Signs and symptoms of potential problems	Fevers, chills, or sweats (persistent) Weight loss (rapid) Cough and increasing shortness of breath and fatigue Increasing fatigue or weakness Nausea, vomiting, diarrhea (frequent and persistent) Pain in chest or abdomen Difficulty swallowing or eating Headaches (increasing and persistent) Visual disturbances (blurring or loss) Numbness, tingling, or burning of the feet or legs Loss of use of a part of the body Sudden changes in mental status or behavior
Medications and treatments	Specific to the medication and treatment
Nutrition	Eat foods high in calories Avoid raw eggs, uncooked meats and fish Clean all vegetables and fruits thoroughly

Source: Adapted from Carr & Gee, 1986.

EXAM QUESTIONS

Chapter 9

Questions 75 - 83

75. When should discharge planning occur?

    a. At discharge
    b. On admission
    c. Several days before discharge
    d. After discharge

76. What scale combines signs and symptoms with activity level to determine functional level?

    a. Gaffky
    b. Columbia Mental Maturity
    c. Karnofsky
    d. Brazelton behavioral

77. During the initial home evaluation, the nurse's assessment of a patient's risk factors is based on information obtained from which of the following?

    a. History and physical examination
    b. Social and dietary history
    c. Inventory of medications
    d. Mental health history

78. The most common signs and symptoms seen in home health nursing of patients with HIV infection or AIDS include:

    a. Fear, mouth ulcers, muscle cramps
    b. Rashes, diarrhea, anxiety
    c. Cough, pain, fatigue
    d. Chills, depression, nausea and vomiting

79. What is one advantage of home health care for patients with HIV disease?

    a. Prevents rehospitalization
    b. Facilitates communication with family members
    c. Provides legal assistance
    d. Reduces cost of medical care

80. Which of the following provides skilled nursing care; social services; home health aides; shopping and meal preparation; and intravenous, respiratory, and physical therapy for patients with HIV disease?

    a. Home health services
    b. Hospital services
    c. Outpatient care
    d. Convalescent care

81. Which of the following involves collaboration with health care providers, patients, and patients' significant others to coordinate hospital, home, and ambulatory care?

    a. Discharge planning
    b. Case management
    c. Outcome criteria
    d. Nursing care planning

82. Lack of communication between care providers and lack of knowledge about community resources are which of the following?

    a. Barriers to discharge planning
    b. Benefits of discharge planning
    c. Barriers to case management
    d. Benefits of home care

83. Which health care systems are coordinated by the case manager?

    a. Clinic, home, and skilled nursing facility
    b. Hospital, home, and skilled nursing facility
    c. Hospital, outpatient care, and home
    d. Home, doctor's office, and rehabilitation center

CHAPTER 10

PSYCHOSOCIAL ISSUES

CHAPTER OBJECTIVE

After studying this chapter, the reader will be able to describe the psychologic and social issues that affect patients with HIV disease, their care providers, and health care workers.

LEARNING OBJECTIVES

After studying this chapter, the reader should be able to

1. Specify the psychosocial issues confronting those with HIV infection and AIDS.

2. Identify the group-specific issues for gay and bisexual men and IDUs who have HIV disease.

3. Recognize the emotional reactions commonly experienced by persons infected with HIV.

4. Indicate the common fears of those who have HIV infection or AIDS.

5. Differentiate between the uncertainties of those with HIV infection and those with AIDS.

6. List the four stages of situational distress that occur in patients who have AIDS.

7. Recognize the common psychologic problems that occur at the time of diagnosis, midstage, and during the terminal phase of illness in a patient with AIDS.

8. Specify what nurses should do if they have prejudices and deep negative feelings about patients who have AIDS.

9. Indicate what group is most at risk when patients with AIDS are hospitalized for care and treatment.

INTRODUCTION

Despite a worldwide campaign of education, widespread and often unreasonable fear still exists about HIV infection, AIDS, and persons who have AIDS. Many patients with AIDS, as well as their families, are still rejected and ostracized. This alienation takes many forms: a lost job, a child kept away from school, a person with visible lesions of Kaposi's sarcoma who is asked to leave an elevator or a restaurant, or once-close relatives who now refuse to visit.

The psychosocial implications of HIV infection and AIDS have been well documented since the syndrome was identified in 1981 (Cassens, 1985; Holland, 1985; Nichols, 1985). The psychologic effects can be catastrophic. The greatest stress is the uncertainty associated with being seropositive. Patients are anxious about their jobs, their family and friends, and their future life.

Several psychosocial features are unique to HIV infection and AIDS (Abrams, Parker-Martin, & Unger, 1989). These include fear of contagion experienced by the public and by the lovers, spouses, family, friends, and workmates of those who have HIV disease; social hostility toward those with the disease who are homosexual or IDUs; lack of traditional family structure among homosexual men and IDUs; and the young age of those infected.

This chapter presents the psychosocial implications of HIV disease. Groups considered include persons with HIV infection and AIDS; their significant others, families, and friends; and their health care providers, especially nurses.

SOURCES OF PSYCHOLOGIC STRESS

HIV disease presents many challenges for adaptation or change during its various stages. The potential for psychologic and social stress is always present. The consequences of being tested for HIV antibodies, a major life-threatening illness, social pressures and disruptions, and reactions to death and dying are major sources of stress. Persons who are seropositive for HIV face changes in life-style and behavior. They must reexamine their priorities and aspirations, cope with complex medical and social systems, and establish adequate relationships with caregivers. Issues once thought resolved must be reconsidered. These include attitudes toward sexuality, dependency needs, reactions to authority figures, and feelings of helplessness (Martin & Vance, 1984; Namir, 1986).

Screening tests for antibodies to HIV can be a major source of stress. Thinking about being tested and about the consequences associated with a positive or negative result creates indecisiveness and fear. Anticipated events may include changes in social behavior and the loss of friends and family.

Persons react in different ways when they find out they are seropositive for HIV. Most become anxious and depressed. They may also feel angry or guilty or think about suicide (O'Dowd & Zofnass, 1991). Some may have a brief, reactive psychosis. Their perceptions of reality are distorted (e.g., they have delusions or hallucinations), and they experience emotional distress.

The social pressures associated with being seropositive create additional stress. Often, those who have HIV disease must deal with loss of job, denial of life and health insurance, eviction, and the effects of adverse legislation. They may be refused police, sanitation, health care, and mortician services (Namir, Wolcott, Fawzy, & Almbaugh, 1987).

Once AIDS has been diagnosed, the uncertainty and anxieties about what will happen are replaced with the uncertainty of how long the person will live and what is going to happen. The loss of jobs and income is an additional stress: How will the patient live and who will provide the necessary health care?

Patients with HIV disease also have social pressures because of their life-style. Maintaining or hiding a gay identity in a hostile heterosexual environment increases stress. Persons who are IDUs face hostility and ostracism in a world that is saying no to drugs. A diagnosis of AIDS forces many drug users to seek detoxification to become drug-free when services are limited or unavailable.

Social pressures also arise from the need for safer sex and drug-using equipment. Religious and social mores may condemn the use of condoms and spermicides. Gay men and IDUs need to develop new coping mechanisms to manage the stresses associated with HIV-related changes in drug-sharing and socializing.

Stress increases as the disease progresses. For someone who is seropositive for HIV, each new sign or symptom causes uncertainties related to the fear of an AIDS diagnosis. Those who have AIDS experience uncertainties about new signs and symptoms and the possibility that any new problem will end in death. Other sources of anxiety are worries about being able to work, obtain enough money to live, and provide self-care.

Table 25 summarizes general and risk-specific issues of patients who have AIDS (Christ, Siegel, & Moynihan, 1988).

Underlying all the psychosocial pressures is the knowledge that death will occur soon. The effects of grief in patients with AIDS and in their friends and

---

Table 25
ISSUES CONFRONTING AIDS PATIENTS

General

- Sharing intimate personal information with health care professionals
- Guilt, shame, and fear
- Interpersonal nature of sex
- Stigma associated with the diagnosis
- Youth or age developmental issues

Gay/Bisexual Men

- Changes in sexual behavior
- Misconceptions of risk and vulnerability
- Dealing with confusion about the value of modifying sexual behavior
- Conflicts between modifications in sexual behavior and efforts to integrate in the homosexual community
- Views of body schema as cause of AIDS
- Cumulative impact of watching numerous friends die of AIDS

Injecting Drug Users

- Specific rituals and ways of interacting within the subculture
- Lack of organized community resources for support
- Many in subculture marginally functional
- Limited ability to cope with stresses of the disease and its treatment
- Effect of addictive drugs on efficacy of pain, depression, antianxiety, and antiemetic medications
- Difficulty complying with treatment programs because of compulsive behavior

Sexual Partners

- Anger
- Disclosure of illness
- Difficulty in caring for children or partner
- Impact of watching spouse, lover, children die of the disease

families have been overlooked by most, especially in areas with the highest numbers of AIDS cases. Grief is frequently the cause of depression, increased use of alcohol and drugs, and withdrawal from normal activities. Persons facing death have a preoccupation with mortality, a sense of personal vulnerability, and heightened emotional distress. Because of this, patients with AIDS may seek multiple opinions from health care providers and try any drug or treatment that may prolong life or cure the disease.

EMOTIONAL REACTIONS TO HIV DISEASE

The most common emotional reactions in patients who have HIV disease are fear, denial, isolation, depression (with thoughts of suicide), anxiety, uncertainty, and guilt (Cassens, 1985; Feinblum, 1986; Holland & Tross, 1985; Morin, Charles, & Malyon, 1984; Salisbury, 1986). Many of these have been mentioned in the preceding paragraphs. Table 26 (p.169) summarizes them.

The psychologic effects of HIV infection and AIDS and adjustment to the stress related to the diagnosis can cause situational distress. The emotional responses are similar to those that occur in any catastrophic event. Classically, situational distress has three stages: initial crisis, transitional state, and deficiency state. In patients with HIV disease, it has four stages: initial crisis, transitional state, deficiency state, and preparation for death (Nichols, 1985; Table 27, p.170).

Many methods have been developed to describe the timing of the emotional reactions. The most common method is to catalogue them according to stage of illness or life cycle. Table 28 (p.171) summarizes the emotional and psychologic problems in patients with AIDS according to the stage of the illness.

Depression and suicide are emotional reactions frequently mentioned but rarely described. Depression is usually related to internalized and unexpressed anger and fear. It is manifested by self-isolation, increased or decreased food intake, abuse of alcohol or drugs, lack of motivation, fatigue, and changes in sleep patterns. Persons who are depressed may not be able to perform normal activities, including activities of daily living. They may also have physical problems. In patients with HIV disease, signs and symptoms normally associated with depression may also be early evidence of ADC. A CT scan of the head and psychologic testing can be used to determine if the signs and symptoms are due to depression or to ADC.

True depression occurs because of the overwhelming fear and anger related to HIV infection. Concerns about the effects of the illness on family, friends, lovers, financial resources, and physical well-being may be so overwhelming that isolation is the only recourse. Anger over being infected; toward the person who caused the infection; or toward society for failure to provide services, treatments, or cures also leads to depression.

In addition, many persons who are chronically depressed are becoming infected with HIV because of their lack of permanent relationships. In an HIV-infected patient who has a primary psychiatric diagnosis of chronic schizophrenia or bipolar personality disorder, depression may intensify. Also, those with unresolved anger as a result of traumatic experiences in childhood and early adulthood may become even more depressed when they find out they are HIV positive.

The estimated rate of suicide among persons infected with HIV is 10–30%, depending on locality. Those who threaten to kill themselves are confronted with feelings of panic, guilt, depression, and hopelessness. Most of those who attempt or succeed at suicide have thought about and discussed the issue with friends or health care providers. Health care

Table 26
SUMMARY OF EMOTIONAL REACTIONS TO HIV INFECTION

Fear of

- Contagion
- Loss of employment, housing, financial support
- Loss of physical attractiveness
- Loss of self-esteem
- Exposure of life-style
- Decreased social support
- Inability to cope
- Increased dependency on others
- Death and dying

Denial of

- Life-style
- Seropositivity to HIV
- Signs and symptoms or illness
- Need for medical or psychologic care
- Need for assistance in activities of daily living

Isolation

- Abandonment by friends, family, lover
- Withdrawal from friends, family, lover
- Refusal to seek available assistance

Depression/Suicide

- Related to anger, fear, isolation
- Concern about ability to manage symptoms and disease progression
- Sadness, helplessness, guilt, worthlessness, hopelessness, social withdrawal, and anticipatory grief

Anxiety

- Severe uncertainty about disease and treatment
- Difficulty setting and maintaining goals
- Severe distress related to new symptoms
- Hypervigilance toward body functions
- Severe uncertainty about others' reactions to the disease or life-style
- Nervousness, insomnia, palpitations, breathlessness, agitation, anorexia
- Repetitive questions
- Continuous thoughts about the disease
- Loss of enjoyment for normal activities and friends
- Immobility or the inability to act on decisions

Uncertainty about

- Disease
- Friends, family, lover
- Treatments
- Employment and financial status
- Future

Guilt about

- Life-style
- Transmission of HIV to others
- Sexual orientation
- Use of drugs

Table 27
EMOTIONAL RESPONSES IN THE FOUR STAGES OF SITUATIONAL DISTRESS

Stage	Response
Initial crisis	Denial
	Fear
	Anxiety
	Anger
	Shock
	Sadness
	Guilt
	Bargaining
Transitional state	Alternating guilt, self-pity, anxiety
	Distress
	Confusion
	Disruptiveness
	Withdrawal
Deficiency state	Formation of new identity
	Acceptance of limitations, illness
Preparation for Death	Fear of dependence
	Completion of unfinished business

Source: Adapted from Nichols, 1985.

providers must be on the alert for potential suicidal ideation and arrange for psychiatric consultation and treatment when needed (Glass, 1988).

Effective intervention with a patient in crisis depends on understanding the patient's current psychosocial stressors. Questioning the patient about perceptions of the source of distress can be both effective and efficient. A question such as, What about your illness is causing you the most stress or discomfort right now? will give insight into what the patient's needs are at the time. Understanding the patient's response will enable the nurse to provide information, reassurance, suggestions, emotional support, or direct care to relieve discomfort. If the patient's needs are resolved first and then nursing is provided, both patient and nurse will have their concerns and needs met.

PSYCHOSOCIAL ASSESSMENT

The psychosocial needs of patients with HIV disease are similar to those of patients who have other chronic or terminal illnesses. Several concepts are useful in making psychosocial assessments. Using these concepts as guidelines for gathering information about a patient will help nurses in two ways.

CHAPTER 10 — PSYCHOSOCIAL ISSUES

Table 28
COMMON PSYCHOLOGIC PROBLEMS ACCORDING TO STAGE OF ILLNESS IN PATIENTS WITH AIDS

Stage of Illness	Problems
Newly diagnosed	Denial, anger Need for financial, emotional, social support Possible impaired self-esteem Fear of treatment Fear of rejection Feelings of guilt, self-blame Changes in life-style (employment, sex, activities)
Mid-stage	Loss of hope Emotional exhaustion Anticipatory loss of independence, important people Anticipation of death Anxiety and fear related to treatments, pain control, comfort Concern and anxiety about unfinished life issues, putting affairs in order
Terminal care	Completion of grief work Anxiety and uncertainty about pain control, personal comfort Concern about interactions with family, friends, lover, spouse Anxiety over wishes relating to death, belongings

Source: Adopted from Dilley, Shelp & Batki, 1986.

They can anticipate the patient's reactions, needs, and vulnerability to potential psychologic dysfunction, and they can plan appropriate interventions.

Psychosocial History

Information about past interpersonal relationships, education, and career will help determine the patient's vulnerability to psychologic dysfunction. Use of nonprescription drugs and alcohol and previous psychiatric care indicate previous psychologic function.

Current Distress and Crisis

Levels of anxiety, fear, and behavioral disorganization are related to the precipitation, duration, and intensity of the crisis experienced by the patient.

Coping

Knowledge about the patient's previous patterns and methods of understanding and resolving problems provides insight and direction. Nurses can use this information to help the patient choose appropriate coping mechanisms.

Social Support

The sources and types of social support available should be assessed. Knowledge of the practical assistance, social interaction, and emotional support available will indicate the types of support and assistance the patient will need.

Life-Cycle Phase

Depending on their age, persons have different resources, skills, goals, and social roles. Most patients with AIDS are in their twenties, thirties, and forties. The developmental task for someone 18–25 years old is intimacy vs. isolation; for someone 25–45 years old, it is generativity vs. stagnation (Erickson, 1963). Illness and dying disrupt these tasks. What is must be reconciled with what might have been.

Illness Phase

Stresses experienced at the time of diagnosis, during treatment, and after treatment differ depending on the clinical syndrome. Emotional reactions and coping responses also differ according to the phase of the illness.

Individual Identity

Sources of self-esteem, goals, valued achievements, orientation to living, and search for meaning affect how patients perceive, face, and battle their illness.

Loss and Grief

The losses the patient has experienced, is experiencing, and will experience affect the type of psychosocial support needed and provided.

Adapted from Flaskerud, 1987, and Wolcott, 1986.

APPROACHES TO HEALING

Nurses have an important role in managing the emotional distress caused by HIV disease. Besides providing direct care, they have a responsibility to provide education, guidance, and emotional support. Patients need to know about the clinical syndrome, treatment interventions, and ways to manage signs and symptoms.

Society's response to HIV disease reflects the cumulative experiences of many individuals. Societal norms frame a person's perceptions and reactions to circumstances. Psychologic adaptation is influenced by medical signs and symptoms; attitudes toward health and illness; premorbid personality; self-concept; previous experience with AIDS; perceptions of the consequence of the disease; and the reactions of family, friends, and society. Nurses can decrease patients' emotional distress by offering ways to understand and relieve rejection and suffering.

One way to reduce anxiety and fear and increase emotional support is to initiate the use of healing elements (McKusick & Tafoya, 1988; Table 29, p.173). These provide the basis for effective treatment of anxiety and other mood disturbances. They also give insight into ways most persons resolve general fear and anxiety. Healing elements enable patients with HIV disease to understand current information about the disease and provide an avenue for reassurance and guidance in resolving the current crisis. They also include qualities of the healer, which must be expressed in a manner respectful of the cultural context of the person who is ill (Pasnau, 1989).

Patients with HIV disease feel guilty and have many fears. They may worry about having their life-style exposed and losing self-esteem and physical attractiveness. They fear death and dying, decreased social

CHAPTER 10 — PSYCHOSOCIAL ISSUES

Table 29
HEALING ELEMENTS IN THE TREATMENT OF AIDS

Power of Naming

With a name, the healer can give an explanatory model in terms of a labeling process available to the patient within the patient's world view.

Punctuation

In many societies, specific rituals, such as marriage, puberty, and widowhood, announce to the community changes in the social status of individual members. In health care, appropriate punctuation, such as starting a drug, creates a possibility of a new, nondiseased state.

Contextualization

The context in which an individual acts shapes the nature of the healing. Persons with HIV disease come from many different cultures and will be healed by health care sensitive to their cultural context.

Group Ritual

Group reality is established through ritual. Group rituals provide a structure for powerful, open expression of emotion in a manner that does not overwhelm individual participants.

Emotional Arousal

Altering the state of the sensorium—the excitement, for example, of faith healing or the somnolence of anesthesia—can open the way to healing. The altered state of emotion can transform the world view and open a hopeful view of the future.

Self-Mastery

Whether by learning a song, ritual, or prayer, by mediation or by structuring or organizing one's life, the individual can increase the sense of personal mastery in response to illness. Skills themselves aid in mastery, but the acquisition of skills is equally empowering.

Personal Qualities of the Healer

The healer's genuineness, warmth, and empathy are critical aspects of the healing process. A sensitive physician will frame concern and action in a language that accommodates the patient's world view.

Source: Adapted from Fullilove, 1989.

---

support and increased dependency, and loss of occupation and financial status. They have concerns and confusion over options for medical treatment and an overriding sense of helplessness associated with a degenerative illness. They face social stigmatization and catastrophic loss. The syndrome reduces social contact, and many patients have already lost significant others or friends to the disease. In addition, some families cannot accept the life-style the patient has lived. Because of this, they are unable to provide emotional and social support (Selwyn, 1986c).

Nurses need to be aware of the psychosocial ramifications of HIV disease. They need to assess interventions and be knowledgeable about the available resources in the community and state so they can make appropriate referrals. They also need to be nonjudgmental and objective. They should provide information and refrain from giving advice. The patient should be allowed to decide which method or treatment or choice is best.

The patient and the patient's family and significant others should have control over activities of daily living and treatments. If a patient or significant others decide to terminate treatments or care, nurses should support them in their decisions. (This does not mean supporting plans for suicide. If a patient or others inform a nurse about an intent to commit suicide, the nurse is obligated to report this information to the physician and to make appropriate intervention to prevent the suicide.)

Patients and significant others should be told the truth about what is happening. If the nurse is not sure what is happening or does not know, this should be made clear also. Information should be given in a way that indicates the reality of the situation while providing some hope. For example, if a patient's condition will lead to death in 1-2 months, the nurse might say, "How long you will live is unknown. It could be a couple of months, or longer." This is better than saying "You have 1 to 2 months." Patients need to be able to trust their health care providers to tell them what they need to know in a timely and appropriate manner.

Finally, nurses should be prepared to listen to each person and provide professional and emotional support through empathy, care, and concern. Time spent listening and sharing with patients is the most significant contribution a nurse can make in their ongoing care. As death approaches, the nurse should not abandon them as many of their friends and families may. Nurses should continue to visit or contact these patients by telephone. This will mean a lot to the patient and any others who are present when death occurs.

NURSING ATTITUDES

Nurses who care for patients with AIDS must have many skills. Because of the intense care demanded, experience with high-dependency or psychiatric nursing and care of patients with terminal illnesses may be helpful. A thorough knowledge of HIV disease, modes of transmission of HIV, and the progressive stages of the illness is essential.

Because so many patients with HIV disease are homosexual or bisexual men or IDUs, knowledge about these groups and their life-styles is important. Nurses must explore and evaluate their own attitudes toward sexual orientation in light of religious and cultural beliefs and societal trends. This is best accomplished by self-questioning and by discussing the issues with close friends, sexual partners, and other nurses.

Nurses should also explore and understand their attitudes toward drug and alcohol use. It is important for nurses to recognize their own reactions to substance abuse. In addition, the number of women with HIV disease is increasing. Nurses must also explore their feelings related to this group.

Some caregivers avoid patients with AIDS because of a tendency to prejudge the patient. Unfortunately, some health care workers still believe that a person with AIDS is somehow getting what he or she deserves. This harks back to early times, when victims of disease were thought to be responsible for their illnesses. Perhaps the many efforts being made to educate everyone about HIV will help change such attitudes.

In some cases, negative feelings about AIDS and patients with AIDS are so strong that they are not easily dispelled. Health care providers who have such feelings need to evaluate and deal with these feelings before they have contact with a patient who has AIDS. All health care professionals must learn to separate personal judgments and beliefs from their professional lives. Perhaps the following sentences from the ANA Code of Ethics (1985), which defines the patient's right to care, are worth reconsidering:

> Patients have a right to be cared for in a manner which respects their human dignity. Refusal to provide care, providing only minimal care, or making derogatory comments to or about the patient are clearly unethical. The rights of the patient and the duties of the nurse are clear.

Even if prejudices about homosexuality or drug use make it difficult for a nurse to deal with a patient with AIDS, the nurse is still required to provide compassionate and respectful care. Nonverbal messages and body language can be quite clear to patients who have AIDS. Therefore, it is important for nurses to settle personal feelings before they attempt to care for a person who has HIV disease.

Can a nurse refuse to care for a patient who has AIDS? A patient with HIV disease presents no greater risk of infection than any other patient with an infectious or life-threatening disease. Because patients with AIDS are often extremely sensitive about the disease and the extensive care required, a nurse's hesitation to provide care or unfounded fears about AIDS will usually be apparent to them. Each health care facility should have specific policies about nurses' refusing to care for patients with certain diseases or conditions. General policy has been that no nurse can refuse to care for a patient because of the patient's disease.

A nurse-administrator who directs an educational outreach program and a training program for nurses who will be treating patients with AIDS has observed that once most nurses get past their initial fears of being infected with HIV, they find that providing care for these patients is no different from working with other patients who have life-threatening diseases. The nurses learn that a patient with AIDS is no more infectious than a person with hepatitis B. They also learn that a patient with AIDS may be more at risk from the persons around him or her than those persons are from the patient (Bennet, 1987).

PSYCHOSOCIAL STRESSORS FOR NURSES AND THEIR FAMILIES

Caring for patients with HIV disease places enormous stresses on health care providers. Nurses are especially prone to these stresses because of the regular and intensive contact they have with patients who have AIDS. Nurses and their families have fears about contagion. Routine contact with patients' body fluids and with contaminated needles and transmission of HIV are constant concerns.

The fear of transmission is also felt by nurses' family members and friends. Family members may place pressure on a nurse to quit because of their fear of the disease. Friends may distance themselves or avoid contact with the nurse altogether.

Discomfort and uncertainty in caring for IDUs and homosexuals place additional stress on the nurse. These patients' backgrounds may challenge the nurse's personal preferences, values, religious ideals, and cultural mores.

For the nurse, the amount of care required by patients with HIV disease is physically and emotionally exhausting. The demands of the patient and the inability to meet the demands of other responsibilities and other patients may increase stress levels. Lack of sufficient support from the institution will also increase emotional and physical exhaustion. The exhaustion is then taken home, where it may affect the nurse's interactions with family members. The result of these stressors is nurse burnout and the eventual loss of the nurse to the profession.

Other matters nurses must contend with are the age of the patients, the sense of personal vulnerability, issues of death and dying, and facing their own mortality. The inability to prolong life conflicts with traditional healing goals. Treatment regimens cause stressful side effects, and patients become debilitated. This in turn creates conflict and ambiguity for the nurse over the need to provide care and comfort. In effect, caring for patients with AIDS challenges the nurse's competency, professional and personal values, and ethical convictions.

A multifaceted program of support is needed to meet the psychosocial needs of nurses who care for patients with HIV disease. This program should include education about HIV infection and AIDS, policies and procedures for infection control, clear goals relating to treatments, emotional support groups, staff meetings, access to mental health consultants, and support from the institution. Supportive measures and guidelines will enable the nurse to provide satisfying care to the patient and will decrease the stressors involved in providing care to patients with HIV disease. Group discussions can foster value and goal clarification, reduce anxiety, and increase emotional and job satisfaction. These discussions should be led by a person who is knowledgeable about the group process, codependency issues, and death and dying.

Nurses may want to develop rituals related to the death of the patient. These might include attending services for the patient, having a special time to remember the patient with other staff members, sending off balloons, or lighting candles. Nurses must allow themselves to grieve over the death of each patient.

Nurses need to take time for themselves when they are dealing with stressful care situations. If they do not care for themselves (taking time off, time out, relaxation time, educational time, meal time), then no one else will either. Nurses who care for themselves are able to better care for their patients.

Together the nurse and the institution can provide for patient and staff support. Acknowledging that stress exists for both groups and providing for stress reduction will enable the nurse and the institution to meet everyone's psychosocial needs.

CONCLUSION

The psychosocial issues related to HIV disease are multiple and complex. They affect the patient, the patient's family and friends, the nurse, the nurse's family and friends, and other health care workers. By understanding the disease better, nurses may be able to provide comprehensive care to help patients with AIDS fight the numerous debilitating conditions that occur. If treatment fails, the nurse can help the patient and the patient's family and friends face death in a calm and peaceful manner. Institutional policies and supportive care will help both the nurse and the patient.

The next chapter discusses ethical and legal issues related to nursing and the care of patients with HIV disease.

EXAM QUESTIONS

Chapter 10

Questions 84 - 90

84. Which of the following encompass fears of contagion, hostility, lack of traditional family structure, and young age of those infected with HIV?

    a. Emotional reactions
    b. Psychosocial issues
    c. Group-specific issues
    d. Common fears

85. What are the most common emotional reactions experienced by persons who have HIV infection?

    a. Anger, hate, fear, and denial
    b. Love, acceptance, peace, and certainty
    c. Fear, denial, isolation, and uncertainty
    d. Apathy, hate, denial, and guilt

86. Which of the following is associated with the transitional state of situational distress in a person with HIV disease?

    a. Shock
    b. Withdrawal
    c. Acceptance of limitations
    d. Fear of dependence

87. What is the difference between the uncertainty of a symptomatic HIV-seropositive person and the uncertainty of a person with AIDS?

    a. Diagnosis of AIDS vs. approaching death
    b. Diagnosis of AIDS vs. disability
    c. Health vs. approaching death
    d. Independence vs. dependence

88. Who is most at risk when a person with AIDS is hospitalized for care and treatment?

    a. The patient
    b. The patient's family and friends
    c. The nurse providing bedside care
    d. The charge nurse

89. Common psychologic problems that occur during the middle stage of illness in patients with AIDS include:

    a. Fear of rejection
    b. Completion of grief work
    c. Need for financial support
    d. Anticipation of death

90. What should nurses do if they have prejudices and negative feelings about persons with AIDS?

    a. Refuse to care for patients who have AIDS
    b. Provide minimal care and infrequent contact
    c. Separate personal and professional beliefs and judgments
    d. Let others know about personal beliefs and judgments

CHAPTER 11

ETHICAL AND LEGAL ISSUES

CHAPTER OBJECTIVE

After studying this chapter, the reader will be able to describe the ethical and legal issues associated with HIV disease and specify the role of nurses who care for patients with ethical and legal problems.

LEARNING OBJECTIVES

After studying this chapter, the reader should be able to

1. Define the term *ethics*.

2. Specify the three areas of ethical study.

3. Discriminate between descriptive, metaethical, and normative ethics.

4. List the five guiding principles of nursing ethics.

5. Specify the most important ethical principle of nursing practice.

6. Differentiate between beneficence and nonmaleficence.

7. Specify a nurse-client interaction that is an example of autonomy.

8. Indicate on what basis the Tarasoff Doctrine is used to inform third parties at risk for HIV infection.

9. Specify the issue or issues related to the ethical principle of justice as applied to AIDS.

10. Specify the meaning of a positive HIV antibody test.

11. Recognize circumstances in which results of a test for HIV antibodies can be released.

12. Indicate who must report a diagnosis of AIDS to the health department and what should be included in the report.

13. Specify why a will is an important legal document for many homosexual and bisexual patients with AIDS.

14. Differentiate between a living will and a durable power of attorney for health care.

15. Select components that should be included in a typical will.

ETHICAL ISSUES

HIV disease presents difficult scientific, ethical, legal, social, and economic challenges to health care providers. It has forced societies to face issues that affect both the general public and persons who are infected. Health care providers and governments have been called on to advance public health and protect those who are disadvantaged and vulnerable (Bayer & Gostin, 1989; Grady, 1989).

Nursing Ethics

Nursing ethics is not a new concern brought about by HIV disease. Since the Florence Nightingale Pledge in 1893, the literature has reflected the breadth and depth of nurses' concern for ethics in practice, education, and society (Fowler, 1989).

Values are the principles on which ethical decisions are based. They are the norms that influence behavior and the ideals each person thinks are important. Nursing professionalism, autonomy, and caring are examples of health care values (Brown, 1987).

Ethics is a philosophical study. It is the descriptive study of morality, the metaethical study of moral judgments, and the normative study of moral problems (Fowler, 1989). Descriptive ethics is the factual description of moral behavior or beliefs. It takes into account real-life situations. Metaethics is concerned with the theoretical issues of meaning and justification. Normative ethics deals with two issues: norms of value and norms of obligation. These are the moral values of "good and evil." Descriptive ethics is the "what is," metaethics is the concern about theories or the "why," and normative ethics is concerned with "what should be or ought to be" (right and wrong).

According to Fowler (1989), ethics provides direction for three types of moral problems:

1. Moral uncertainty: Doubt about moral principles or rules that may apply, or the nature of the ethical problem.

2. Moral dilemma: A conflict of moral principles that support different ways in which to act.

3. Moral distress: Knowledge of the right action to take but inability to take it because of institutional constraints.

Normative ethics is the discipline that has guided nursing practice. Within this discipline, nursing uses the analytical model for decision making. This model relies on deductive application of rules and principles, which can be specified in many ways. Five of these principles are respect for persons, autonomy, beneficence and nonmaleficence, fidelity, and justice (Fowler, 1989; Grady, 1989). These five are contained in the Code for Nurses established by the ANA.

The most important principle and first obligation of nursing practice is respect for persons. Some have maintained that this broad principle is the supreme moral principle from which all ethical principles and rules are derived. Respect for persons "means that we treat ourselves and others with a respect inherently due humans and that we recognize, in a moral sense, that we all share a common human destiny" (Fowler, 1989, p. 959).

The derivative principle of autonomy makes the principle of respect for persons applicable to nursing practice. Autonomy is a person's right to control his or her life as long as no harm is done to others (Fowler, 1989). Autonomy in nursing practice is translated into advocacy of patients. As advocates, nurses show respect for their patients' wants and needs. Advocacy indicates that the nurse will take or has taken appropriate action to fulfill these needs or wants. Acting as an advocate shows respect for patients' autonomy and enables them to make choices. Nurses have a responsibility to be advocates and to ensure patients' autonomy.

In health care, beneficence and nonmaleficence are usually combined and considered as one ethical principle. The combined principle has four aspects: not inflicting harm (nonmaleficence), removing harmful conditions (beneficence), preventing harm (beneficence), and positively benefiting another or doing good (beneficence) (Fowler, 1989).

Beneficence is the principle that governs the nurse's obligation to provide care. By entering the profession, nurses have obligated themselves to do no harm to the patient and to promote the good of the patient. The codes of ethics of the ANA and the International Council of Nurses make it unacceptable for a nurse to refuse to care for a patient because of the patient's personal attributes, politics, economic status, or illness (Grady, 1989). The only exception is when the nurse's physical, emotional, or other wellbeing is threatened.

Nursing fidelity encompasses both autonomy and confidentiality. Confidentiality is the assurance, trust, or reliance that all information about a person (patient) is private and personal. It is based on respect for the individual. The principle of fidelity symbolizes a moral obligation to keep commitments and promises made to others.

Some of the most pressing issues today concern health care resources and access to health care. These are related to the principle of justice. Commitment to health care systems and society's moral obligation to provide some level of health care to each of its members are issues raised because of this principle.

HIV Infection and Nursing Ethics

Nurses are in a position to confront HIV infection in an ethical and rational manner. They are also in a position to model ethical behavior toward persons infected with HIV and toward sound and just public policies related to HIV infection. The five principles of ethics give direction to interaction with and care of HIV-infected patients. The following paragraphs address each principle as it applies to HIV infection and AIDS.

Persons infected with HIV and their families and friends have a right to be treated with respect and dignity. The guiding principle here is autonomy. Examples of actions related to this principle in nursing practice are advocacy for patients and the doctrine of informed consent. By acting as an advocate, the nurse ensures that patients with HIV infection have adequate information and opportunities to make informed decisions and to make their wants and wishes known. Nurses educate patients, start discussions about HIV disease, and enable patients to make decisions. Areas involved include informed consent, directives related to legal and medical matters, and decisions about advance directives (Grady, 1989).

In order to give informed consent, patients must be provided with sufficient information to make a decision, and they must be free of internal or external influences so that the decision is regarded as free participation. In addition, they must be competent to make a decision (Fowler, 1989; Grady, 1989). Nurses can actively participate by making assessments of the patient's mental competence, providing general information, and clarifying data already obtained by the patient. They should also ensure that patients are given the most accurate, up-to-date information available about HIV disease, procedures, and treatments (benefits and adverse effects) in an environment that is free of coercion or manipulation. Discussions about health care, treatment choices, and advance directives should occur as early as possible to avoid concerns about mental competency. Nurses show respect when they provide the patient opportunities to think about, discuss, and plan for difficult decisions about life support.

Advance directives are documents related to future care, treatment, research, and life-sustaining therapies. They include the living will, durable power of attorney, durable power of attorney for health care, wills, and the designation of a proxy if mental incompetence should occur. These documents are used to indicate the patient's person of choice, the person who will act on the patient's behalf if needed. They are important for someone who is a lover, friend, or family member of a patient with HIV disease. Without a legal document giving them permission, the persons of choice have nothing to safeguard their participation in making decisions about the patient's care and other matters (Grady, 1989).

Most controversial ethical decisions in medical care are related to the right to life or the right to death. Decisions about starting or stopping life-sustaining procedures are easier if they are discussed and made before such procedures are needed. Decisions may include both written and oral statements about sustaining life when cardiac or respiratory arrest or brain death occurs. Because legal documents vary from state to state and hospital to hospital, nurses should be aware of the legal requirements in their state and hospital. When the decision to terminate care or life support is controversial, the ability of a family or individual to make the decision should be reviewed by an institution-based ethics committee.

The nurse's responsibility to provide care and to prevent harm or harmful conditions is an application of the principle of beneficence. Refusing to provide care, providing only minimal care, and making derogatory comments to or about the patient are violations of this principle. Refusing to provide care is usually based on statements that caring for the patient would be harmful to the nurse because of the possibility of transmission of HIV. The risk of acquiring HIV infection in the work environment is minimal (less than 0.035%). Refusing to care for a patient because of the risk of becoming infected is not justifiable.

Nonmaleficence is the principle of not inflicting harm. From a nursing perspective, this includes not only physical harm but also emotional, psychologic, spiritual, and moral harm. Both the sanctity and the quality of life of patients with HIV disease are protected by this principle. Quality of life must be determined by the patient, not by the nurse or other health care providers. Quality for one person may not be quality for another. For both nurses and patients, values clarification is important in carrying out this principle.

The issue of confidentiality regarding HIV infection and AIDS is an ongoing controversy. Although all states require that cases of AIDS be reported, each state has different regulations about reporting cases of HIV infection. Information about a person's status with regard to AIDS and HIV infection is a sensitive and complex issue.

Confidentiality is an ethical requirement of health care professionals. Patients share a large amount of private and sensitive information about themselves and their families. Disclosure of this or of information on HIV infection without the patient's consent can have dire results. Patients may face discrimination and isolation. Losses of jobs, housing, and insurance have occurred. Children infected with HIV have been prevented from attending school or participating in after-school activities. Children with HIV disease have been abandoned by their parents because the parents could not accept the child's life-style or were afraid of becoming infected (Fowler, 1989; Grady, 1989).

Confidentiality, however, is not an absolute. Laws about disclosure of a patient's HIV status vary from state to state. Most states now have laws that allow disclosure of HIV status to an at-risk partner or to a third party under certain conditions. It has been argued that telling a person's sexual partners that the person is seropositive for HIV is justifiable. The reason is the risk to the sexual partners' health. This argument is based on the Tarasoff Doctrine. This doctrine defines the duty of a therapist as the responsibility to provide reasonable protection to an intended victim of crime (homicide or suicide). Protection implies notification of the potential victim, the police, or any others. The Tarasoff Doctrine has been invoked in arguing that health care workers must notify the sexual or needle-sharing partners of a patient who is seropositive in order to protect the partners' lives (Bayer & Gostin, 1989; Melton, 1988).

Who should inform the sexual or needle-sharing partner is also a controversial issue. In most cases, the person who is infected is expected to tell the partner(s). If the person refuses or does not tell the partner(s), then the physician or health care provider should do the informing. A patient's refusal or failure to inform partners should be carefully documented, along with the response of the person informed.

Controversy also exists over the right of health care providers to know the serologic status of patients. This includes testing of hospitalized patients and informing other health care providers about the results. Some institutions permit informing others within the institution but not outside it. Some states have laws that permit informing other health care providers when the patient's care or life is at risk or when the health care provider's life is at risk.

The issue is difficult to resolve because risk (patient and personal) is the reason most health care providers seek to know a patient's serologic status. Insufficient or unknown information about a patient could affect the nurse's ability to provide appropriate and timely care. Knowing that a patient is seropositive for HIV enables the nurse to plan for care and teach and support the patient, the patient's family and friends, and other members of the nursing staff (Grady, 1989).

Access to health care resources and services is an issue related to the principle of justice. In many situations, persons infected with HIV do not have equitable access to health care services. Physicians, nurses, and others have refused to provide care and services to patients with HIV disease. Discharge planning and placement in long-term care facilities can be difficult. Residential and day-care facilities and foster homes have refused to admit patients with HIV disease. Many of those infected are poor and disadvantaged and did not have adequate care and services before they became infected. Patients who are homeless have additional problems because it is difficult to obtain benefits without an address (Grady, 1989).

Financial resources for care of the poor and homeless have always been inadequate. The added burden of HIV disease has strained already overstretched services. As health care providers, nurses are challenged to provide resources and services despite limited funds. Nurses can offer many services in nonhospital settings, which would improve access and increase quality of care. They can also be advocates for services and care through the legislative process and by applying for grants. Finally, nurses are collectively a large voting bloc with a potentially powerful lobby that can influence changes in health care legislation, regulation, and delivery (Grady, 1989).

LEGAL ISSUES

Many of the legal issues facing patients with HIV disease are similar to the ethical issues. Breaches in ethical practices frequently lead to discrimination, loss of confidentiality, and lack of respect. Nurses should be aware of at least three general legal areas: confidentiality, consent, and estate planning. Both legal and ethical issues are involved in confidentiality; informed consent; power of attorney; suicidal or homicidal ideation; and choices regarding treatment, scope of care, loyalty, and life support.

Consent to Testing and Confidentiality

Written consent should be obtained before a person's blood is tested to detect antibodies to HIV. The only exceptions to this are (1) when state laws permit testing without permission in special circumstances (i.e., rape or offenses against law officers) or (2) when the person cannot give consent and someone else (i.e., a conservator) is given permission to grant it. Nurses should be knowledgeable about laws in their state and local area on who can give consent.

A consent form, signed by the patient, is used only when the test is required for reasons other than checking donated blood. A separate form, "The Blood Donor Information Form," is used by blood banks and plasma centers. This form includes medical information. If it is to be used in the hospital, it should be reviewed first and approved by the appropriate medical staff committee or the designated physician.

The laws, rules, and regulations on consent for HIV antibody testing vary among states and institutions. Nurses should know what the laws, rules, regulations, and policies are for their state and health care institution. In general, a person may not be tested for HIV antibodies without giving consent. Consent can be verbal. However, most lawyers agree that consent for HIV testing should be in writing and should follow the general guidelines for informed consent.

The person being tested must receive counseling before consent is given and the test is done and again after the test is completed, regardless of the results. Results of HIV testing should always be given in person. The results should never be given over the telephone or to someone other than the person who had the test. Those who do the counseling and give the person tested the results should be familiar with the meaning and implications of the results.

Counseling is an important component in preventing the transmission of HIV. Information about their serologic status may help persons who are not infected make changes in their behavior that will reduce their risk of becoming infected. Persons who are seropositive may be encouraged to make changes that will prevent the transmission of HIV to others.

Counseling should include the information on the following:

- Specificity and sensitivity of the test
- Meaning of positive and negative tests
- Transmission of HIV
- How to prevent transmission of HIV
- Confidentiality
- Recording of the results in the medical record (indicate if the records will have a copy of the results and where the results will be recorded)
- Community resources

Counseling serves two purposes. First, it explains the test and its purpose so the person can make a decision based on current information. Second, it is an effective means of providing education on HIV infection, transmission of HIV, and prevention of transmission.

A positive result on the enzyme-linked immunosorbent assay (ELISA) does not mean that the person has AIDS. It does means that the person has been infected with HIV at some time in the past and that antibodies to the virus have developed. In addition, a positive results on an ELISA must be confirmed by results on either a Western blot test or another confirming test. Positive results on both Western blot and ELISA indicate infection with HIV and development of antibodies. Because the long-term prognosis of HIV infection is still unknown, counseling services should be available for those who do not have AIDS, and long-term follow-up and support should be provided and encouraged.

Those whose test results are negative should be informed that they may still be infected with the virus. In some instances, the tests are done before the anti-

CHAPTER 11 —
ETHICAL AND LEGAL ISSUES

bodies to HIV have developed. These persons should be counseled to abstain from or avoid behaviors that put them at risk and to have the test repeated in 3–6 months.

Results of tests to detect antibodies to HIV are confidential. Disclosure of the information in any way that identifies the patient is strictly limited. Disclosure includes all releases, transmissions, disseminations, or communications, whether they are made orally, in writing, or electronically. Each separate disclosure must be authorized by the patient. Disclosure without written consent may result in a penalty.

A valid authorization to disclose results of tests for antibodies to HIV must be in writing, and it must specify the person to whom the disclosure will be made. In addition, the authorization may stipulate that the results can be disclosed only by a person who is responsible for the care and treatment of the person who had the test.

Because of the deadly nature of HIV disease, the long-standing rules of confidentiality between patient and physician or nurse are being challenged on many fronts. Balanced against the patient's right to privacy and confidentiality is the danger of spread of infection to the patient's sexual partner, children, and health care personnel. Several states as well as the federal government have established laws governing notification of the patient's sexual partner(s). All nurses should be aware of these laws in their state. In addition, the American Medical Association (AMA) adopted a statement urging physicians to notify third parties of a patient's HIV status (AMA, 1988).

The AMA recommends a three-part process in notifying partners of a patient's serologic status:

1. The physician should try diligently to get the patient to notify the third party or parties.

2. If that fails, the physician should report the matter to state or local health authorities, requesting that they assume responsibility. Some states are now equipped to handle such responsibility; others are not.

3. If the state refuses the case or is unable to notify the third party, then the physician must handle notification personally.

Many of the behaviors associated with transmission of HIV are private and personal. Education designed to cause changes in these behaviors requires sensitivity and discretion. Counseling should include information on transmission of HIV, information on behaviors that put a person at risk, strategies to reduce risks, emotional-psychologic exploration of problem areas and strengths, and recommendations for personal health behaviors (McMahon, 1988).

General Principles of Confidentiality

The following two general principles of confidentiality may be helpful for those who are not involved in counseling for HIV testing.

1. Each separate disclosure must have written authorization. The results of tests for HIV are confidential. Disclosure in any way that identifies the patient is strictly limited. In addition, the authorization may state that the results can be disclosed only by a person who is responsible for the care and treatment of the person who had the test. Separate written authorization is required for each disclosure of the test results.

2. Unauthorized disclosure may result in a penalty. Willful or negligent disclosure of the results of a test for antibodies to HIV or of the identification of the person to whom the test results apply will lead to penalties in many states. Penalties apply only if the disclosure is not authorized by the patient or by

law. They do not apply when the information is disclosed in order to meet reporting requirements for a diagnosed case of AIDS to the state health department or to the CDC.

Nurses should review their state's regulations and the testing and confidentiality guidelines of their hospital or institution. Each is a little different, but nearly every health care group has guidelines for confidentiality of patient records.

Mandatory Reporting of a Diagnosis of AIDS

Since June 1985, all physicians and hospitals are required to report immediately all transfusion-related AIDS cases (as confirmed by the person responsible for caring for the patient with AIDS) to the county health officer for investigation. In addition, all health care providers are required to report each case of AIDS to the CDC. If a patient is hospitalized, the hospital reports the case. If the diagnosis is made in a clinic or private physician's office, then the clinic or office must make the report.

Special report forms have been developed by the CDC for reporting of a case of AIDS. However, if the forms are not available at the time, the report should include the following: the patient's name, address, telephone number, birth date, social security number, and risk behaviors; AIDS diagnosis; date of diagnosis; and the names of the reporter and reporting facility and person.

Epidemiologic and clinical information on patients with AIDS is reported to the CDC in Atlanta by state and local health departments. A standard confidential case report form is used. The mean interval between diagnosis of an AIDS case and notification of the CDC is 2 months (CDC, 1989a).

ESTATE MATTERS

Financial planning is important for patients with AIDS because of the length of the illness and the medical costs incurred (Robertson, 1983). Patients need to plan for this care as best as they can. Up to 73% of patients with AIDS become incapacitated or die within 2 years of the diagnosis. Because of this, wills and other documents should be drawn up as soon as possible.

An unmarried couple, particularly a homosexual couple, has special legal problems. The partner of a deceased or incapacitated gay person, even a lifelong partner, has none of the rights and protections the law affords legally married spouses. Thus, the patient's wishes may be ignored unless documents are legally executed before the patient becomes incapacitated or before death occurs. Depending on the assets involved, the persons who need to be protected, and other considerations, a patient who has AIDS should consider several legal avenues with the help of a lawyer.

Joint Ownership or Joint Tenancy

A patient with AIDS may want to consider establishing joint ownership of property or assets, or may want to review such arrangements if they already exist. For example, the patient may want to make sure property is not still owned jointly with a former lover. Bank accounts can be easily converted to joint ownership, which will give the lover or family member ready access to funds. This might be important if someone other than the patient will need to take charge of the funds during the patient's lifetime. (The same result can be achieved through a power of attorney.) If the funds in the bank are less than $30,000, placing them in a joint account will facilitate distribution to the surviving joint owner after the patient's death.

CHAPTER 11 —
ETHICAL AND LEGAL ISSUES

Trusts

An *inter vivos* trust can be useful for patients with HIV disease who are currently capable of managing their business affairs but who may become incapacitated. This document allows the lover or a trusted friend to manage the patient's assets in the event the patient becomes incapacitated and avoids the need for a conservator. It also allows the trustee to immediately manage the patient's assets without obtaining a court order.

Powers of Appointment

A lover or trusted friend may be given authority to act on behalf of the patient. Powers of appointment have been used to grant authority to a designated lover or friend to make medical decisions if the patient is unable to do so. Another suggestion is that hospital questions about next of kin not be answered by the patient at the time of admission. This is an appropriate alternative for patients who have a poor relationship with their next of kin and for patients who prefer to have contact only with a lover or other close friends when hospitalized. If the hospital or primary physician is advised that the patient has no next of kin, the desires of family or relatives will not be brought to bear during the illness.

Conservators

Patients might also be encouraged to designate a conservator or guardian in the event they become incapacitated. This can be accomplished with a simple document and will prevent much unhappiness, particularly if the patient has hostile family members whose appointments to conservatorships would not be in the patient's best interests. A lover or other trusted friend is a good candidate for this type of appointment.

Conservatorship is a statutory mechanism by which the court appoints a person to assist another who has become incapacitated and needs help managing assets and/or personal care. Such a conservator is appointed by the court on the petition of a relative, friend, or anyone who believes, in good faith, that he or she is acting in the best interests of the patient.

The terms and limitations of conservatorships vary by state. However, two types of conservatorship or guardianship are generally used. The first is a conservatorship for the estate. With this type, the conservator is legally responsible for managing the patient's assets and financial affairs. The second type is a conservatorship for the person. With this type, the conservator is responsible for making sure the patient's needs for health, food, clothing, and shelter are met. Patients with AIDS may need both types of conservatorships. Court approval is necessary for most actions taken by the conservator and thus can be costly. The patient's attorney can consider alternatives such as the *inter vivos* trust or power of attorney. Even if these are used, the patient will need to execute a written and witnessed nomination of conservator, which will prevent appointment of a blood relative, which occurs in most states.

Durable Power of Attorney

A durable power of attorney is another means of protecting patients who might become mentally or physically incapacitated. Two types are available: general and medical or health care. The traditional power of attorney goes into effect when the person issuing the document becomes disabled. The durable power of attorney authorizes another person to make decisions on the first person's behalf even after disability occurs. The durable power of attorney for health care can authorize another person to make decisions after the death of the person who issues the document. The documents extend many powers to the patient's legal representative. Not all states have a durable power of attorney for health care. In such cases, if the patient wants someone other than a biological family member to make medical decisions, the patient should sign a separate document authorizing the designated agent to make such decisions.

This written authorization can be persuasive when dealing with a physician, especially when the patient's intent is clear.

The Patient Self Determination Act

The (federal) Patient Self Determination Act went into effect January 1, 1992. This law requires health care facilities, home health agencies, hospices, and prepaid programs such as health maintenance organizations to provide information and education about advance directives. This education and information is to be given to patients, staff personnel, and the community.

Advance directives are legal documents executed by patients to have their wishes related to feeding, resuscitation, and care carried out if they should become legally incompetent or disabled. The most common documents are durable power of attorney, durable power of attorney for health care, directives to physicians, and living wills. Nurses need to understand the rights, obligations, and the legal liabilities related to these documents.

Patients should be provided an opportunity to execute such documents. Once the document is executed, it should be given to those who are mentioned in the document and placed in all medical records. The medical record should flagged or marked to indicate that such a document exists (Markus, 1991).

All nurses must become informed about these directives and about the new law. Additional information should be available in the workplace or from local nurses' associations.

Living Wills

A living will is a written directive to the family, physicians, and other health care providers made while a patient is competent. It expresses the patient's desire to have medical treatment halted if the patient becomes incompetent and unable to request that treatment be stopped. Active euthanasia is illegal, even if the person is suffering greatly. A living will gives the physician who relies on the directive immunity from civil and criminal liability for withholding care.

The statement directing the physician to remove life-support systems must be precise, and it must conform to the rigid requirements of the statutes of the state where it is executed. The living will must be written to the patient's physician by the patient. Additional written evidence of the patient's intention may be helpful if the patient's lover or a friend asks that the physician remove life-support systems and the patient's family is opposed to this. In addition to giving the physician a copy of the exact living will form, patients with HIV disease may want to write a letter to their physician expressing their wishes before they have a serious decline in health.

It is helpful for patients to reexecute their living will every 5 years, so that it reflects their current thinking, even if this is not required by state law. In addition, they should enlist the help of a close relative or friend who will act as their advocate and ensure compliance with the living will when they enter the hospital.

In states that have no provisions for living wills, patients may want to write one anyway, in the hope that their wishes will be followed. Living wills may be legally binding in states that do not have legislation on them.

A living will can be revoked at any time, even if the patient's competency at the time is in question. The will can be revoked by burning, tearing, canceling, or obliterating the document or by signing a witnessed and notarized statement that it is revoked. Most states also allow oral revocation.

Wills

For patients who wish to leave all or a portion of their estate to someone other than a biological family member, a will is essential. Each state has its own statutes that prescribe who shall inherit the assets of someone who dies without making a will (intestate). A will should be drawn up even when other documents have been designed to dispose of the patient's estate, such as in a trust. This will help avoid legal battles if the other documents are lost or invalidated. A will serves as further evidence of the patient's intent and may cover items that might have been inadvertently omitted in other documents.

A simple will has four basic ingredients:

1. The testator's name and address.

2. Directions on disposition of the body.

3. The names of the beneficiary or beneficiaries (disposition of property). (An alternative beneficiary should be named in case the first beneficiary dies before the testator or dies in a common accident with the testator.)

4. The executor's name and address. (An alternative should also be chosen.)

Homosexuality is usually irrelevant to the will when no other grounds exist for contesting it. Generally, an attorney will discuss the legal implications of a will to help allay the patient's fear that the will might be contested.

If a patient is terminally ill or in a weakened mental or physical state when the will is drawn, the family may contest it, claiming the will was drawn while the patient was mentally incapacitated or under undue influence. In situations in which the patient's lover is the beneficiary, the attorney should make sure the lover is not present when the will is discussed or signed, because this may create the appearance of undue influence. The attorney should also document the patient's capacity at the time the will is signed.

If there is a possibility that any person might contest the will as an heir, such as a spouse, child, or grandchild, a statement of specific omission must be placed in the will.

Selecting an Executor

Patients should be advised to select an executor, such as a friend or institution, who is reliable and competent to carry out the administration of their estate. Several successors or alternatives should also be named. In addition, it is often a good idea to give one or more of the nominees the power to nominate a coexecutor, alternative, or successor.

It is particularly important for patients with AIDS who are gay to have documents that clearly state what they want done with their body. Such documents may prevent painful clashes between a patient's biological family and a lifelong partner over where the deceased should be buried. In many cases, family members have prevented the partner from seeing the patient after death and then have taken the body away for burial or cremation.

Some patients with HIV disease may resist making funeral or burial plans because of the nature of the disease or because they hope to survive until a cure is found or because of denial. In such cases, these patients may be far more comfortable having another specified person—whether a lover or a family member—handle the arrangements when the time comes ("Constitutional Rights of AIDS Carriers," 1986).

CONCLUSION

Ethical and legal issues related to HIV disease pose multiple challenges for health care professionals, particularly nurses. The ability of the nurse to confront risks and remain impartial while providing care and services will make a difference for patients and the patients' family and friends as they cope with this terminal illness. The ability of an institution to meet the needs of both patients and staff members will determine the effectiveness of providing services to this group.

EXAM QUESTIONS

Chapter 11

Questions 91 - 100

91. What is the philosophical study of morality, moral problems, and judgments?

    a. Descriptive ethics
    b. Metaethics
    c. Ethics
    d. Normative ethics

92. What are the three areas of ethical study?

    a. Descriptive ethics, metaethical ethics, and normative ethics
    b. Moral behavior, moral problems, and normative ethics
    c. Moral judgments, metaethical ethics, and morality
    d. Morality, descriptive ethics, and normative ethics

93. What area is concerned with theories or the "why" of ethics?

    a. Descriptive ethics
    b. Moral values
    c. Metaethics
    d. Moral dilemmas

94. What ethical principle is being practiced when a nurse permits an HIV patient to determine whether treatment is continued or stopped?

    a. Fidelity
    b. Justice
    c. Autonomy
    d. Respect for persons

95. Under what circumstances may the results of HIV testing be revealed to another party?

    a. With verbal consent of the person tested
    b. With written consent of the person tested
    c. With an order from a court of law
    d. When an HIV-positive patient is referred from one physician to another

96. What doctrine is being invoked when a health care provider informs a pregnant woman that her sexual partner is seropositive for HIV?

    a. Monroe
    b. Tarasoff
    c. Religious
    d. Governmental

97. The right of persons with HIV infection to have equal access to health care resources and services is an issue related to which ethical principle?

    a. Respect for persons
    b. Autonomy
    c. Fidelity
    d. Justice

98. What is the meaning of a positive result on a test for antibodies to HIV?

   a. The person will die within 6 months.
   b. The person has AIDS.
   c. The person is not infected with HIV.
   d. The person is infected with HIV.

99. Which of the following statements about a living will and a durable power of attorney for health care is correct?

   a. A durable power of attorney does not take effect until after the death of the patient.
   b. A living will provides physicians immunity from civil or criminal liability for withholding health care.
   c. A living will must be written by the patient.
   d. A durable power of attorney must be executed every 2 years.

100. Which of the following are required by law to report each case of AIDS to the Centers for Disease Control?

   a. Laboratory technicians
   b. Emergency medical technicians
   c. HIV test sites
   d. Health care providers

This concludes the final examination. An answer key will be sent with your certificate so you can determine which of your answers were correct and incorrect.

APPENDIX

HIV TESTING IN FLORIDA

In 1988, the Florida Legislature addressed the issues associated with acquired immune deficiency syndrome (AIDS) for the first time. It recognized that AIDS is transmitted by a retrovirus, which makes the possibility of discovering an immunization or cure in the near future highly unlikely and which means that an individual, once infected, has a high probability of developing the disease and dying prematurely. The Legislature further recognized that public fears about AIDS had affected the attitudes of employers, insurers, educators, law enforcement personnel, and health and medical providers about dealing with those individuals stricken with the disease. Thus, it acted to create a balance between medical necessity, the right to privacy, and protection of the public from harm. The result was a series of statutes to establish programs for the care and treatment of persons with AIDS and related conditions, and to set parameters for testing to detect human immunodeficiency virus (HIV) infection and AIDS in individuals. This article will address the testing, confidentiality, and treatment guidelines established by the Florida Legislature.

It is important to remember that the laws regarding HIV testing, treatment, and reporting are somewhat fluid. As yet, few Florida courts have interpreted the provisions of these statutes. Thus, while the information provided here is current as of April 1993, it is subject to ongoing amendment, clarification, and refinement by the courts and the Legislature.

Having concluded that the public health would be served by facilitating informed, voluntary, and confidential use of tests designed to detect AIDS and HIV infection, the Florida lawmakers enacted Section 381.004 of the Florida Statutes to provide guidelines for human immunodeficiency testing. As a general rule, testing for the HIV virus, or its antigen or antibody[1], may not be performed without the informed consent of the individual to be tested ("test subject"). Informed consent, as used in this context, contemplates that, at a minimum, the person upon whom the test is to be performed be given an explanation of the confidential status which attaches to both the test subject and the test results. In addition, the test subject must be provided with information about how a person can be exposed to HIV, how the virus is transmitted, and how HIV infection can be prevented. At the time the test is ordered, a return visit must be scheduled for face-to-face disclosure of the test results. Note, consent need not be in writing provided there is documentation in the individual's record that the test has been explained and consent has been obtained. Section 381.004(3)(a), (c), Florida Statutes (1991).

The statute further provides that when the tested individual returns for his results, he must be afforded the immediate opportunity for individual counseling about the meaning of the results, the possible need for further testing, measures for preventing transmission of the virus, and the availability in the individual's geographic area of appropriate health care services, mental health care, and social and other support services. The individual must also be advised of the benefits of locating and counseling any other person who may have exposed the patient to the virus or any person whom the test subject may have exposed, plus the availability, if any, of public health assistance to locate and counsel those other persons. Section 381.004(3)(e), Florida Statutes (1991).

---

1 The statute and guidelines relate not just to tests that are currently adminstered, but to all HIV-related tests as they are developed and become available.

The Florida Legislature provided some exceptions to this rule. Informed consent by the person to be tested is not required in some circumstances. For example, an HIV test may be performed in the case of a medical emergency where the test results are necessary for diagnostic purposes in order to provide appropriate medical care or treatment to the person being tested, even if the patient is unable to consent. All of the foregoing must be documented in the patient's medical record, and post-test counseling, described above, is required. HIV testing may also be performed for diagnostic purposes where, in the opinion of the attending physician, obtaining informed consent would in some way be detrimental to the patient. Again, the circumstances must be documented in the patient record, and post-test counseling must be made available if the counseling would not be detrimental to the patient. The statute clearly states, however, that these exceptions are not intended to authorize the routine testing of patients without first obtaining informed consent. Section 381.004(3)(i)(3), (4), Florida Statutes (1991).

Another exception exists for the testing of persons accused of sexual battery. The victim of a sexual offense is entitled to know whether the person charged with the offense is HIV positive. The victim, or the victim's parent or legal guardian, may request that the accused undergo HIV testing. The results of that testing must be disclosed to the accused and may also be disclosed, upon request, to the victim or the victim's parent or legal guardian[2]. Section 960.003, Florida Statutes (1991).

An exception also exists with respect to health care providers. These individuals (referred to in the statutes as "medical personnel") may request that an HIV test be performed on a patient for whom they are caring, without the patient's consent, if the health care provider has been subjected to a "significant exposure" during the course and scope of the provider's employment. In this context, significant exposure means exposure to blood or body fluids through needle stick, instruments, or sharps, or exposure of mucous membranes or skin to visible blood or body fluids to which universal precautions apply. Included in this category are blood, semen, vaginal secretions, cerebral spinal fluid, synovial fluid, pleural fluid, peritoneal fluid, pericardial fluid, amniotic fluid, or laboratory specimens that contain HIV. Health care providers who can make this request include licensed or certified health care professionals; employees of health care professionals, health care facilities, or blood banks; paramedics; and emergency medical technicians. Section 381.004(2)(c), 3(f)(12), Florida Statutes (1991).

The circumstances under which an HIV test can be performed at the request of a health care provider, without the patient's consent, exist in two separate sets of facts. The first occurs where a blood sample has been taken from the patient voluntarily for other purposes such as routine blood testing performed for diagnostic reasons. Prior to conducting the requested HIV test, the patient must be asked to consent to the performance of the test and release of the results. Should the patient refuse to consent, that refusal, plus any additional information concerning the performance of the test and the test results, is to be documented in the health care provider's record rather than in the patient's medical record.

If consent is not obtained because the patient cannot be located, reasonable attempts to locate him must be made and the attempts must be documented prior to performing the tests. If the patient does, in fact, refuse to consent to the test, he must be informed that the test will be performed anyway, and counseling, discussed previously, must still be provided to him. Note that under this set of facts there is no provision for requiring a patient to give a blood sample in the face of the patient's refusal to do so. Therefore, if no blood has already been obtained prior to the health care provider's request, the test cannot be performed without the patient's consent. Section 381.004(3)(i)(10), Florida Statutes (1991).

The second set of facts that would permit a health care provider to request that an HIV test be performed on a patient without the patient's consent occurs where the health care provider has been subjected to a significant exposure during the course and scope of his employment while he is providing emergency medical treatment

---

[2] Att least one Florida court has ruled that the person charged with a sexual offense has no correlative right to compel the victim to be tested for HIV. *State v. Brewster*, 601 So. 2d 1289 (Fla. 5th DCA 1992).

to the patient. In that case, the tests may be performed only during the course of the patient's treatment for the medical emergency[3]. Many of the requirements in this scenario are identical to those in the first set of facts above. An attempt must be made to obtain informed consent from the patient. Any refusal to consent, plus information concerning the test and its results, are to be documented in the health care provider's records. Section 381.004(3)(i)(11), Florida Statutes (1991).

In either scenario, the test may be conducted only after a licensed physician documents, in the medical record of the health care provider, that there has been a significant exposure and that, in the physician's medical judgment, the information is medically necessary to determine the course of treatment for the health care provider. Moreover, the health care provider cannot compel testing of an individual unless the health care provider is first tested for HIV or provides the results of an HIV test taken within six months prior to the significant exposure. Section 381.004(3) (i)(10), (11), Florida Statutes (1991).

The emergency medical treatment exception also applies to nonmedical personnel who provide emergency medical assistance during a medical emergency occurring outside of a hospital or other physician-staffed health care facility. As in the case of health care providers, a physician must document in the nonmedical personnel's medical record that there has been a significant exposure and that the information is medically necessary. The nonmedical personnel must also provide documentation of HIV testing before the patient can be compelled to undergo the test. Section 381.004(3)(i)(11), Florida Statutes (1992 Supp.).

With few exceptions, both the identity of any person upon whom HIV testing has been performed and the test results are confidential, and no person who has obtained or has knowledge of a test result may disclose, or be compelled to disclose, the identity of a test subject or the results of a test. Persons and entities who may obtain the otherwise confidential information include: persons, including insurers, whom the test subject designates in a legally effective release; health care providers consulting between themselves or with health care facilities to determine diagnosis and treatment; health care facilities or health care providers that procure, process, distribute, or use human body parts from deceased persons or semen provided prior to July 1988 for the purpose of artificial insemination; employees of health care facilities who participate in the provision of patient care or who handle or process specimens of body fluids or tissues, where the employee has a need to know such information; and health care providers, discussed above, who have been subjected to a significant exposure during the course and scope of their professional duties. Section 381.004(3)(f), Florida Statutes (1991).

In addition, hospitals and other licensed facilities have an obligation to notify emergency medical technicians, paramedics, or other persons transporting sick or injured patients to those facilities if they have come into direct contact with a patient who is subsequently diagnosed as HIV positive. The facility must, however, notify the emergency medical technician, paramedic, or other person transporting the patient in such a way that protects the patient's confidentiality and does not disclose the patient's name. Section 395.0147, Florida Statutes (1992 Supp.).

An exemption to the rule against disclosure of HIV test results also exists with respect to physicians, under certain conditions. Where a patient who has tested positive for HIV discloses to his physician the identity of his or her sexual or needle-sharing partner(s), the physician may recommend that the patient notify his or her partner(s) and refrain from sexual or drug activities likely to transmit the virus. If the patient refuses, the physician may advise the partner(s) of the patient's positive HIV test results. He must first inform the patient of his intention to do so, and the disclosure must be reasonable and in good faith, pursuant to a "perceived civil duty" or ethical professional obligation. While the statute relieves a physician from civil or criminal liability

---

3   Medical emergency, although not defined for purposes of HIV testing guidelines, is defined elsewhere in the Florida Statutes as a medical condition manifesting itself by an acute symptom of sufficient severity, including severe pain, that, without immediate medical attention, could reasonably be expected to result in serious jeopardy to the patient's health, serious impairment to bodily functions, or serious dysfunction of any bodily organ or part. Section 395.0142 (2) (c), Florida Statutes (1991).

for disclosing HIV test results without the patient's consent, it does not impose any duty on the physician to notify a patient's sexual or needle-sharing partners, and relieves him from civil or criminal liability if he fails to so inform those individuals. Section 455.2416, Florida Statutes (1991).

Notwithstanding the provision that informed consent for HIV testing must be obtained from a parent or legal guardian of a minor, a minor can consent to examination and treatment for sexually transmittable diseases, including AIDS, without the consent of his or her parents or guardian. It would appear, therefore, that minors can consent to HIV testing without parental consent, providing that such testing is performed as a part of a more comprehensive examination and/or course of treatment for AIDS or other sexually transmitted disease. As with adults, the fact of consulting, examining, or treating the minor is confidential and cannot be divulged, subject to the exceptions previously described. To protect that confidentiality, the testing or treating provider is prohibited from sending a bill for those services to the minor's parent or guardian without the consent of the minor. Section 384.30, Florida Statutes (1991).

Florida Statutes provide that it is unlawful for any facility or person licensed by the Agency for Health Care Administration, the Department of Health and Rehabilitative Services, or the Department of Professional Regulation to require any person to submit to HIV testing as a condition of admission to the facility or of obtaining service. It does not, however, prohibit any physician in good faith from declining to provide a particular treatment requested by a patient if the appropriateness of that treatment can only be determined through an HIV test. In other words, if the physician believes that the treatment which a patient has requested should only be performed in the absence (or presence) of HIV, the physician may require that the patient submit to an HIV test to determine the absence (or presence) of HIV. If the patient refuses to submit to the test, the physician may refuse to perform the requested treatment. Section 381.004(11), Florida Statutes (1992 Supp.).

Finally, Florida law requires that any health care facility or provider that conducts a testing program for AIDS, AIDS-related complex, or HIV must provide face-to-face pre- and post-test counseling. The pre-test counseling must inform the test subject of the meaning of a test for HIV, including medical indications for the test. It must advise of the possibility of false-positive or false-negative results and the potential need for confirmatory testing. The program must also provide counseling on the potential social, medical, and economic consequences of a positive test result, and on the need to eliminate high-risk behaviors. Much of the same information must be provided in the mandated face-to-face post-test counseling. Individuals who provide post-test counseling as part of the testing program are required to receive specialized training about the special needs of persons with positive results, including recognition of possible suicidal behavior. In addition, patients must be referred for further health and social services as appropriate. Section 381.004(5), Florida Statutes (1991).

CONCLUSION

In the areas of HIV testing, treatment, and reporting, Florida lawmakers have attempted to balance the differing, and sometimes competing, interests of the patient, the health care provider, and the public. As a general rule, HIV tests may not be performed on an individual without that person's informed consent, and the results of such testing are confidential and may not be revealed to anyone but the tested individual. In practice, however, that rule does not always meet the needs of the people it was intended to benefit, and exceptions, discussed above, have been created. The laws continue to evolve as circumstances require and as the public's attitudes toward persons with HIV and AIDS change.

(1992) Bonnie Eyler, R.N., M.S.N., J.D. and Vanessa A. Reynolds, J.D.
Revised (1993) Vanessa A. Reynolds, J.D.

GLOSSARY

Acquired immune deficiency syndrome (AIDS): a group of tumors or diseases that indicate an underlying cellular immunodeficiency in a person who did not have an underlying immunodeficiency, who has not received medications that could cause immunosuppression, and who did not previously have a malignant tumor. It is the end stage of an ongoing infection with the human immunodeficiency virus (HIV). The syndrome is diagnosed by specific criteria established by the Centers for Disease Control and Prevention (CDC).

AIDS-related complex (ARC): the old term for symptomatic HIV disease; signs and symptoms that appear after clinical latency in a person infected with HIV and before the appearance of any AIDS-defining illness. These may include persistent lymphadenopathy; a decrease in the number of CD4 cells; weight loss; loss of an immune response to skin tests for such things as mumps virus, *Candida*, and tetanus toxoid; fever; night sweats; fatigue; lethargy; rashes or skin lesions; thrush; oral hairy leukoplakia; and changes in the complete blood cell count.

Antibody: a protein formed by the body in response to a foreign substance (antigen), such as measles virus, mold, dust, medications, and foods. Each antibody is specific for the antigen that caused its formation.

Antigen: a substance foreign to the body that causes the formation of antibodies.

Antigenemia: the presence of a foreign substance in the bloodstream.

Antiviral: any drug that can destroy or weaken a virus.

Bacterium (pl. bacteria): a microscopic organism composed of a single cell. Some bacteria can cause disease in humans.

B cell: a type of lymphocyte involved in the production of antibodies. Activated B cells differentiate to form plasma cells, which produce antibodies. A part of the immune system.

Biopsy: the surgical removal of a piece of tissue from a living subject for microscopic examination of the cells in the tissue.

Candidiasis: an infection caused by the fungus *Candida albicans*. It can affect the skin, mucous membranes, and internal organs.

CD4 cell: see T helper cell.

CD8 cell: see T suppressor cell.

Cell-medicated immunity: a type of immunity mediated by cells rather than by antibodies. It requires the coordinated activity of helper and suppressor T cells.

Cofactor: a factor other than the basic causative agent of a disease that increases the likelihood that disease will develop. Cofactors may include the presence of other microorganisms or infections, drugs, alcohol, nutrition, stress, rest or activity, and genetic factors.

DNA (deoxyribonucleic acid): a nucleic acid found chiefly in the nucleus of living cells that is responsible for transmitting hereditary characteristics and is necessary for reproduction or replication.

Diagnosis: identifying a disease by its signs, symptoms, course, and by laboratory findings.

Drug resistance: the ability of an microorganism to resist or withstand the effects of a drug that are lethal to most members of its species.

ELISA: enzyme-linked immunosorbent assay. An ELISA is used to detect antibodies to HIV. A positive result along with positive results on a confirmatory test indicates a person has been infected with HIV.

Epidemiology: the study of the incidence, distribution, environmental causes, and control of a disease or an occurrence in a population. Examples of occurrences are automobile accidents, smoking, and alcohol use.

Epstein-Barr virus (EBV): a herpeslike virus that causes one kind of mononucleosis. It has also been associated with Burkitt's lymphoma, a cancer of the lymph glands.

Etiology: the study of the causes and origins of diseases and their occurrence.

Genome: the genetic endowment of an organism.

Hairy leukoplakia: benign white plaques on the lateral aspect of the tongue, which cannot be removed.

Helper/suppressor ratio: the ratio of helper T cells to suppressor T cells. The normal helper-to-suppressor ratio is approximately 2 to 1 (2:1). In persons infected with HIV, the ratio is inverted; the person has more suppressor than helper T cells.

Hemophilia: a rare, hereditary bleeding disorder of males, inherited through the mother, caused by a deficiency in the ability to make one or more blood-clotting proteins.

Hepatomegaly: abnormal enlargement of the liver.

Herpes simplex virus (HSV): a herpesvirus that causes oral (cold sores) or genital infections characterized by the formation of small vesicles or blisterlike areas on the skin, often around the lips, nose, or genital or perineal areas.

Herpes zoster virus (HZV): also called varicella-zoster virus; a herpesvirus that causes chickenpox (varicella). After the initial infection, the virus can become dormant in the nerves of the spinal column and later cause a disease called shingles (herpes zoster).

High-risk behaviors: a term used to describe certain activities that increase the risk of contracting infections or diseases. For HIV, these behaviors include oral, vaginal, or anal intercourse without a condom and sharing of intravenous needles and syringes that have not been cleansed.

Human immunodeficiency virus (HIV): the virus that causes HIV disease.

HIV disease: a spectrum of disease that begins with HIV infection and ends with AIDS. A person may be infected with HIV for many years before showing signs and symptoms of infection and before progression to AIDS occurs.

Humoral immunity: the human defense mechanism that involves the production of antibodies.

Immune system: the body system that functions as the natural defense mechanism. This system helps the body resist or eliminate disease-producing microorganisms and other foreign substances.

Incubation period: the time between initial infection and the first signs or symptoms of the disease.

In vitro: within glass, observable within an artificial environment. A cell that reproduces itself in the laboratory is said to have reproduced in vitro.

In vivo: within a living organism.

Kaposi's sarcoma: a tumor of the walls of blood vessels that appears as pink-to-purple spots on the skin or internal organs.

Latency: a period when a virus or other microorganism occupies the body but is in an inactive or dormant state.

Lesion: any abnormal change in tissue because of injury or disease.

Lymphadenopathy: swollen, firm, and possibly tender lymph nodes that occur because of infection or cancer.

Lymph node or lymph gland: the body tissue made up of lymphocytes and connective tissue that produces lymph and lymphocytes. Lymph nodes filter impurities from the body.

Lymphoma: a malignant growth of the lymph nodes.

Macular: a discolored or thickened skin eruption that is flat or flush with the skin.

Morbidity: the rate of diseases, accidents, or illnesses, usually expressed as incidence or prevalence.

Mortality: the rate of death from diseases, accidents, or illnesses at a particular time or place.

Opportunistic infections: diseases caused by microorganisms commonly present in the environment or the body; the organisms cause disease only when a change in the normal, healthy condition of the body leads to a weakening or impairment of the immune system.

Orthostatic hypotension: the abnormal lowering of the blood pressure when a person stands; also known as postural hypotension.

Pancytopenia: an abnormal condition in which the numbers of all blood cells are markedly reduced, including white cells, red cells, and platelets.

Papular: a small, solid, raised discoloration or thickening of the skin.

Pathogen: any disease-producing microorganism.

Pyramidal tract signs: an objective finding resulting from involuntary or reflex movement of the muscles. The pyramidal tract consists of a group of fibers in the white matter of the spinal cord that conduct motor impulses down through the anterior horn cells from the opposite side of the brain, causing voluntary and reflex activity of the muscles.

Retrovirus: a class of viruses that contains the genetic material ribonucleic acid (RNA). These viruses must occupy a host cell and convert their RNA into DNA in order to replicate. The process is mediated by reverse transcriptase.

Reverse transcriptase: an enzyme produced by retroviruses that is used by the infected host cell to produce a DNA copy of the viral RNA.

Seroconversion: the point at which antibodies to specific antigens become detectable in the blood.

Splenomegaly: abnormal enlargement of the spleen.

Syndrome: a group of symptoms and signs that occur together and characterize a particular disorder or disease.

T cell: a type of lymphocyte that is formed in the thymus and is part of the immune system.

T helper cell: (also known as T4 cell or CD4 cell) A subset of T cells that is the master regulator of the body's immune system. It is the primary target of HIV.

T suppressor cell: (also known as T8 cell or CD8 cell) A subset of T cells that helps counter foreign agents invading the body and shuts off the formation of B cells and T cells.

Thrush: abnormal, whitish, cheesy exudate of the mucous membranes and skin caused by the fungus *Candida albicans*

Tumor: a swelling or enlargement that may be benign or malignant.

Unsafe sex: see high-risk behaviors.

Varicella-zoster virus (VZV): see herpes zoster virus.

Vesicle: a thin-walled, raised area of the skin containing fluid; a blister.

Virus: a microorganism that invades cells and alters their chemistry so the cells are compelled to produce more virus particles.

Western blot test: a test used to detect antibodies to specific proteins. It is more specific than ELISA for HIV and is considered a confirmatory test for positive results on ELISA. It detects a reaction to proteins specific to HIV.

BIBLIOGRAPHY

Abrams, D. I., Dilley, J. W., Maxey, L. M., & Volberding, P. A. (1986). Routine care and psychosocial support of the patient with acquired immunodeficiency syndrome. Medical Clinics of North America, 70, 707–720.

Abrams, D. I., Parker-Martin, J., & Unger, K. W. (1989). Psychosocial aspects of terminal AIDS. Patient Care, 23, 41–60.

The advent of combination antiretroviral therapy. (1991, August). HIV Frontline, p. 5.

AIDS poses dilemma for doctor-patient confidentiality. (1988, August). AIDS Alert, pp. 1–2.

AIDS Project/LA. (1986). Living with AIDS: A self-care manual. Los Angeles: Author.

Allen, J. R., & Setlow, V. P. (1991). Heterosexual transmission of HIV: A view of the future [Editorial]. Journal of the American Medical Association, 266, 1695–1696.

AMA House of Delegates. (1988). Statement on partner notification. Chicago: American Medical Association.

American Foundation for AIDS Research. (Spring 1992a). d4T. AIDS/HIV Treatment Directory, 5(4), 27, 94.

American Foundation for AIDS Research. (Spring 1992b). *Pneumocystis carinii* pneumonia. AIDS/HIV Treatment Directory, 5(4), 71.

American Foundation for AIDS Research. (Spring 1992c). MAC (*Mycobacterium avium* complex). AIDS/HIV Treatment Directory, 5(4), 63–66.

American Nurses' Association. (1985). Code for nurses with interpretive statements. Kansas City, MO: Author.

Amodio-Groton, M. (1992). HIV drug interactions. AIDS Clinical Care, 4, 25–29.

ANA statements focus on HIV issues. (1991, November/December). American Nurse, 23(10), 24–27.

Are investigational drugs moving through system too slowly? (1988, January). AIDS Alert, pp. 1, 3.

Aronow, H. A., Brew, B. J., & Price, R. W. (1988). The management of the neurological complications of HIV infection and AIDS. AIDS, 2(Suppl. 1), S151–S159.

Arpadi, S., & Caspe, W. B. (1990). Diagnosis and classification of HIV infection in children. Pediatric Annals, 19, 409–420.

Azithromycin update. (1991). PAAC Notes, 3, 201–203

AZT therapy for early HIV infection. (1990). Clinical Courier, 8(5), 1–8.

Bakermann, L. (1988). An overview of antiviral therapy. In G. P. Wormser (Ed.), AIDS: Acquired immune deficiency syndrome and other manifestations of HIV infection: Epidemiology, etiology, immunology, clinical manifestations, pathology, control, treatment, and prevention (pp. 158–176). New York: Alfred Noyes.

Bartlett, J. G. (1992). 1992–1993 recommendations for the medical care of persons with HIV infection. Critical Care America, Baltimore.

Bartlett, J. G., Laughon, B., & Quinn, T. C. (1988). Gastrointestinal complications of AIDS. In V. T. DeVita, Jr., S. Hellman, & S. A. Rosenberg (Eds.), AIDS: Etiology, diagnosis, treatment, and prevention (2nd ed., pp. 227–244). Philadelphia: Lippincott.

Bayer, R., & Gostin, L. (1989). Legal and ethical issues in AIDS. In M. S. Gottlieb, D. J. Jeffries, D. Mildvan, A. J. Pinching, T. C. Quinn, & R. A. Weiss (Eds.), Current topics in AIDS (Vol. 2, pp. 263–286). New York: Wiley.

Beaver, B. L., Hill, J. L., Vachon, D. A., Moore, V. L., Hines, S. E., Seiden, S. W., Stone, M., Hutton, N., & Johnson, J. P. (1990). Surgical intervention in children with human immunodeficiency virus infection. Journal of Pediatric Surgery, 25, 79–84.

Becker, C. E., Cone, J. E., & Gerberding, J. (1989). Occupational infection with human immunodeficiency virus (HIV). Annals of Internal Medicine, 110, 653–656.

Being Alive. (1991, October). Women and HIV/AIDS: Special report (pp. 3, 6). San Diego: Author.

Bennett, J. A. (1987). Nurses talk about the challenge of AIDS. American Journal of Nursing, 87, 1150–1155.

Bernstein, L. J., Mackenzie, R. G., Oleske, J. M., & Pizzo, P. A. (1989). AIDS in children and adolescents. Patient Care, 23, 80–114.

Berry, R. K. (1988). Home care of the child with AIDS. Pediatric Nursing, 14, 341–343.

Brennan, T. (1991). Transmission of the human immunodeficiency virus in the health care setting: Time for action. New England Journal of Medicine, 324, 1504–1509.

Brew, B., Rosenblum, M., & Price, R. W. (1988). Central and peripheral nervous system complications of HIV infection and AIDS. In V. T. DeVita, Jr., S. Hellman, & S. A. Rosenberg (Eds.), AIDS: Etiology, diagnosis, treatment, and prevention (2nd ed., pp. 185–197). Philadelphia: Lippincott.

Brown, M. L. (1987). AIDS and ethics: Concerns and considerations. Oncology Nursing Forum, 14(1), 69–73.

California Nurses Association. (1987). Nurses coalition on AIDS care plan for persons with AIDS: AIDS resource manual (Appendix B). San Francisco: Author.

Carpenito, L. J. (1983). Nursing diagnosis: Application to clinical practice. Philadelphia: Lippincott.

Carr, G. S., & Gee, G. (1986). AIDS and AIDS-related conditions: Screening for populations at risk. Nurse Practitioner, 11(10), 25–48.

Carr, G. S., & Marin, M. M. (1988). Mycobacterial diseases in HIV infection. In G. Gee & T. A. Moran (Eds.), AIDS: Concepts in nursing practice (pp. 165–176). Baltimore: Williams & Wilkins.

Carr, G. S., Newlin, B., & Gee, G. (1988). AIDS-related conditions. In G. Gee, & T. A. Moran (Eds.), AIDS: Concepts in nursing practice (pp. 104–122). Baltimore: Williams & Wilkins.

Carter, S. K., Glatstein, E., & Livingston, R. B. (1982). Principles of cancer treatment (p. 22). New York: McGraw-Hill.

Carter, W. A., Strayer, D. R., Brodsky, I., & Lewin, M. (1987). Clinical immunological and virological effects of ampligen, a mismatched double-stranded RNA, in patients with AIDS or AIDS-related complex. Lancet, 1, 1286–1292.

Cassens, B. J. (1985). Social consequences of the acquired immunodeficiency syndrome. Annals of Internal Medicine, 103, 768–771.

Castro, K. G., Hardy, A. M., & Curran, J. W. (1986). The acquired immunodeficiency syndrome: Epidemiology and risk factors for transmission. Medical Clinics of North America, 70, 635–649.

CDC reports few. (1992, January/February). Nurseweek/California Nursing, p. 27.

Centers for Disease Control. (1981). Pneumocystis pneumonia, Los Angeles. Morbidity and Mortality Weekly Report, 30, 250–252.

Centers for Disease Control. (1982). Kaposi's sarcoma and pneumocystis pneumonia among homosexual men, New York City and California. Morbidity and Mortality Weekly Report, 30, 305–308.

Centers for Disease Control. (1985a). Education and foster care of children infected with human T-lymphotrophic virus type III/lymphadenopathy-associated virus. Morbidity and Mortality Weekly Report, 34, 517–521.

Centers for Disease Control. (1985b). Recommendations for assisting in the prevention of perinatal transmission of human T-lymphotrophic virus type III/lymphadenopathy-associated virus and acquired immunodeficiency syndrome. Morbidity and Mortality Weekly Report, 34, 721–732.

Centers for Disease Control. (1985c). Recommendations for preventing transmission of infection with human T-lymphotrophic virus type III/lymphadenopathy-associated virus in the workplace. Morbidity and Mortality Weekly Report, 34, 681–695.

Centers for Disease Control. (1986a). Acquired immunodeficiency syndrome, United States. Morbidity and Mortality Weekly Report, 35, 757–766.

Centers for Disease Control. (1986b). Classification system for human T-lymphotrophic virus type III/lymphadenopathy-associated virus infections. Morbidity and Mortality Weekly Report, 35, 334–339.

Centers for Disease Control. (1986c). Immunization of children infected with human T-lymphotrophic virus type III/lymphadenopathy-associated virus. Morbidity and Mortality Weekly Report, 35, 595–606.

Centers for Disease Control. (1986d). Recommendations for preventing transmission of infection with human T-lymphotrophic virus type III/lymphadenopathy-associated virus during invasive procedures. Morbidity and Mortality Weekly Report, 35, 221–223.

Centers for Disease Control. (1987a). Classification system for human immunodeficiency virus (HIV) infection in children under 13 years of age. Morbidity and Mortality Weekly Report, 36, 225–230.

Centers for Disease Control. (1987b). Human immunodeficiency virus infections in health-care workers exposed to blood of infected patients. Morbidity and Mortality Weekly Report, 36, 285–289.

Centers for Disease Control. (1987c). Recommendations for prevention of HIV transmission in health-care settings. Morbidity and Mortality Weekly Report, 36(Suppl. 2S), 3S–12S.

Centers for Disease Control. (1987d). Revision of case definition for AIDS for surveillance purposes. Morbidity and Mortality Weekly Report, 36(Suppl.), 1S–8S.

Centers for Disease Control. (1988). Universal precautions for prevention of transmission of human immunodeficiency virus, hepatitis B virus, and other bloodborne pathogens in health-care settings. Morbidity and Mortality Weekly Report, 37, 377–387.

Centers for Disease Control. (1989a). Cases of specific notifiable diseases—United States. Morbidity and Mortality Weekly Report, 38, 738.

Centers for Disease Control. (1989b). Guidelines for prophylaxis against *Pneumocystis carinii* pneumonia in persons infected with human immunodeficiency virus. Morbidity and Mortality Weekly Report, 38(Suppl. S5), 1–9.

Centers for Disease Control. (1989c). Recommendations for treating HIV-infected children. Morbidity and Mortality Weekly Report, 38(13), 205.

Centers for Disease Control. (1990a). Acquired immunodeficiency syndrome—United States. Morbidity and Mortality Weekly Report, 39, 81–86.

Centers for Disease Control. (1990b). Public Health Service statement on management of occupational exposure to human immunodeficiency virus, including considerations regarding zidovudine postexposure use. Morbidity and Mortality Weekly Report, 39, RR-1.

Centers for Disease Control. (1991a). Acquired immunodeficiency syndrome—United States, 1981–1990. Morbidity and Mortality Weekly Report, 40, 357–364.

Centers for Disease Control. (1991b). Guidelines for prophylaxis against *Pneumocystis carinii* pneumonia for children infected with human immunodeficiency virus. Morbidity and Mortality Weekly Report, 40(RR-2), 1–13.

Centers for Disease Control. (1991c). The HIV/AIDS epidemic: The first 10 years. Morbidity and Mortality Weekly Report, 40, 357–364.

Centers for Disease Control. (1991d). Recommendations for preventing transmission of human immunodeficiency virus and hepatitis B to patients during exposure-prone invasive procedures. Morbidity and Mortality Weekly Report, 40(RR-8), 1–9.

Centers for Disease Control. (1992a). AIDS statistical information as of November 30, 1991. Medline, Computer Information Service.

Centers for Disease Control. (1992b). Cases of selected notifiable disease, United States, week ending December 21, 1991, and December 22, 1990 (51st week). Morbidity and Mortality Weekly Report, 40, 894, Table II.

Centers for Disease Control. (1992c). 1993 revised classification system for HIV infection and expanded surveillance case definition for AIDS among adolescents and adults. Morbidity and Mortality Weekly Report, 41(RR-17), 1–20.

Centers for Disease Control National AIDS Clearinghouse. (1992, December 3). Pediatric AIDS cases reported. Rockville, MD, 1-800-458-5231.

Chaisson, R. E., McCutchan, J. A., Nightingale, S., Young, L. S. (1993). Managing *Mycobacterium avium* complex infection. AIDS Clinical Care, 5, 1–8.

Chaisson, R. E., & Slutkin, G. (1989). Tuberculosis and human immunodeficiency virus infection. Journal of Infectious Diseases, 159, 96–100.

The changing demographics of AIDS patients. (1991). PAAC Notes, 3, 183.

Christ, G. H., Siegel, K., & Maynihan, R. T. (1988). Psychosocial issues: Prevention and treatment. In V. T. DeVita, Jr., S. Hellman, & S. A. Rosenberg (Eds.), AIDS: Etiology, diagnosis, treatment, and prevention (2nd ed., pp. 321–337). Philadelphia: Lippincott.

Clark, C. (1990, June 23). Some people infected with AIDS virus might escape the disease. San Diego Union, p. A3.

Clark, C. (1992, November 28). New found hopes for tots born with HIV. San Diego Union, pp. A1, A15.

Clement, M., & Hollander, H. (1992). Natural history and management of the seropositive patient. In M. A. Sande & P. A. Volberding (Eds.), The medical management of AIDS (3rd ed., p. 91). Philadelphia: Saunders.

Clinical use of hyperthermia. (1990). In summary of site visit report. Unpublished manuscript.

Clumeck, N., Van de Perre, P., Carael, M., Rouvroy, D., & Nzaramba, D. (1985). Heterosexual promiscuity among African patients with AIDS. New England Journal of Medicine, 33, 182.

Coffin, J. M. (1990). The virology of AIDS: 1990. AIDS, 4(Suppl. 1), S1–S8.

Cohen, P. T., Sande, M., Volberding, P. A. (1990). The AIDS knowledge base. Waltham, MA: Medical Publishing Group.

Connor, E. (1991). Advances in early diagnosis of perinatal infection. Journal of the American Medical Association, 266, 3474–3475.

Constitutional rights of AIDS carriers. (1986). Harvard Law Review, 99, 1274–1292.

Conte, J. E., Hollander, H., & Golden, J. A. (1987). Inhaled or reduced-dose intravenous pentamidine for *Pneumocystis carinii* pneumonia: A pilot study. Annals of Internal Medicine, 107, 495–498.

Cotton, D. J., & Friedland, G. H. (1992). Case Watch. AIDS Clinical Care, 4, 61.

Crocker, K. S. (1989). Gastrointestinal manifestations of the acquired immunodeficiency syndrome. Nursing Clinics of North America, 24, 395–406.

Crumpacker, C. S. (1988). Treatment of opportunistic viral infections. AIDS, 2(Suppl. 1), S191–S193.

Curran, J. W. (1985). The epidemiology and prevention of the acquired immunodeficiency syndrome. Annals of Internal Medicine, 103, 657–662.

Dannemann, B., Israelski, D. M., Remington, J. S. (1988). Treatment of toxoplasmic encephalitis with intravenous clindamycin. Archives of Internal Medicine, 148, 2477–2482.

DeLoughry, T.J. (1991, December 4). 40 scientists call on colleagues to re-evaluate AIDS theory. Chronicle of Higher Education, pp. A9, A14–A15.

DeVita, V. T., Jr., & Hellman, S. (1982). Hodgkin's disease and the non-Hodgkin's lymphoma. In V. T. DeVita, Jr., S. Hellman, & S. A. Rosenberg (Eds.), Cancer principles and practice of oncology (pp. 1331–1401). Philadelphia: Lippincott.

DeVita, V. T., Jr., Hellman, S., & Rosenberg, S. A. (Eds.). (1985, 2nd ed. 1988; 3rd ed. 1992). AIDS: Etiology, diagnosis, treatment, and prevention. Philadelphia: Lippincott.

Dhundale, K., & Hubbard, P. M. (1986). Home care for the AIDS patient: Safety first. Nursing 86, 16, 34–38.

Dilley, J. W., Shelp, E. E., & Batki, S. L. (1986). Psychiatric and ethical issues in the care of patients with AIDS. Psychosomatics, 27, 562–566.

Drew, W. L., Buhles, W., & Erlich, K. S. (1988). Herpesvirus infections (cytomegalovirus, herpes simplex virus, varicella zoster virus): How to use ganciclovir (DHPG) and acyclovir. Infectious Disease Clinics of North America, 2, 495–509.

Epidemiologic aspects of the current outbreak of Kaposi's sarcoma and opportunistic infections. (1982). New England Journal of Medicine, 301, 248–252.

Epstein, L. G., Goudsmit, J., Paul, D. A., Morrison, S. H., Connor, E. M., Oleske, J. M., & Holland, B. (1987). Expression of human immunodeficiency virus in cerebral spinal fluid of children with progressive encephalopathy. Annals of Neurology, 21, 397–401.

Erice, A., Jordan, M. C., Chace, B. A., & Fletcher, C. (1987). Ganciclovir treatment of cytomegalovirus disease in transplant recipients and other immunocompromised hosts. Journal of the American Medical Association, 257, 3082–3087.

Erickson, E. (1963). Childhood and society. St. Louis: Mosby.

Etheridge, P., & Lamb, G. S. (1989). Professional nursing case management improves quality, access and costs. Nursing Management, 20(3), 30–35.

Eyster, M. E., Goedert, J. J., Sarngadharan, M. G., Weiss, S. H., Gallo, R. C., & Blattner, W. A. (1985). Development and early natural history of HTLV antibodies in persons with hemophilia. Journal of the American Medical Association, 253, 2219–2223.

Fahrner, R., & Nelson, W. J. (1988). Protozoal diseases in HIV infection. In G. Gee & T. A. Moran (Eds.), AIDS: Concepts in nursing practice (pp. 141–164). Baltimore: Williams & Wilkins.

Falloon, J., Eddy, E., Roper, M., & Pizzo, P. A. (1988). AIDS in the pediatric population. In V. T. DeVita, Jr., S. Hellman, & S. A. Rosenberg (Eds.), AIDS: Etiology, diagnosis, treatment, and prevention (2nd ed., pp. 339–351). Philadelphia: Lippincott.

Falloon, J., & Masur, H. (1992). Infectious complications of HIV: *Pneumocystis carinii* pneumonia and other protozoa. In V. T. DeVita, Jr., S. Hellman, & S. A. Rosenberg (Eds.), AIDS: Etiology, diagnosis, treatment, and prevention (3rd ed., pp. 157–167). Philadelphia: Lippincott.

Fauci, A. A. (1991). Optimal immunity to HIV: Natural infection, vaccination, or both. New England Journal of Medicine, 324, 1733–1735.

FDA approval of fluconazole (FDA notes). (1990). PAAC Notes, 2, 76–79.

FDA: Drug approval procedures speeded. (1988, October 20). Los Angeles Times, pp. 1–4.

Fegan, C. (1992). Cryptosporidial disease in the adult HIV-infected patient. Journal of the Association of Nurses in AIDS Care (JANAC), 3(4), 11–20.

Feinberg, J. (1992, January). Using foscarnet: Practical considerations. AIDS Clinical Care, p. 5.

Feinblum, S. (1986). Pinning down the psychosocial dimensions of AIDS. Nursing & Health Care, 71, 255–257.

Fineberg, H. V. (1988, October). The social dimensions of AIDS. Scientific American, 259(4), 128–134.

Fischl, M. A. (1988). Treatment and prophylaxis of *Pneumocystis carinii* pneumonia. AIDS, 2(Suppl. 1), S143–S150.

Fischl, M. A. (1992). Treatment of HIV infection. In M. A. Sande & P. A. Volberding (Eds.), The medical management of AIDS (3rd ed., pp. 97–110). Philadelphia: Saunders.

Fischl, M. A., Dickinson, G. M., & LaVoie, L. (1988). Safety and efficacy of sulfamethoxazole and trimethoprim chemoprophylaxis for *Pneumocystis carinii* pneumonia in AIDS. Journal of the American Medical Association, 259, 1185–1189.

Fischl, M. A., Dickinson, G. M., Scott, G. B., Kimas, N., Fletcher, M. A., & Parks, W. (1987). Evaluation of heterosexual partners, children, and household contacts of adults with AIDS. Journal of the American Medical Association, 257, 640–644.

Fischl, M. A., Richman, D. D., Grieco, M. H., & Gottlieb, M. S. (1987). The efficacy of azidothymidine (AZT) in the treatment of patients with AIDS and AIDS-related complex: A double-blind, placebo-controlled trial. New England Journal of Medicine, 317, 185–191.

566 receives treatment IND. (1991). PAAC Notes, 3, 203–204.

Flaskerud, J. H. (1987). AIDS: Psychosocial aspects. Journal of Psychosocial Nursing, 25(12), 9–16.

Flaskerud, J. H. (1989). Overview: AIDS/HIV infection and nurses' needs for information. In J. H. Flaskerud (Ed.), AIDS/HIV infection: A reference guide for nursing professionals (pp. 1–13). Philadelphia: Saunders.

Flaskerud, J. H., & Ungvarski, P. J. (1992). HIV/AIDS: LA guide to nursing care (2nd ed.). Philadelphia: Saunders.

Follansbee, S. E., Busch, D. F., Wofsy, C. B., Coleman, D. L., Gullett, J., Aurigemma, G. P., Ross, T., Hadley, W. K., & Drew, W. L. (1982). An outbreak of pneumocystis pneumonia in homosexual men. Annals of Internal Medicine, 96 (Part I), 705–713.

Fowler, M. D. (1989). Ethical decision making in clinical practice. Nursing Clinics of North America, 24, 955–965.

Friedland, G. H., & Klein, R. S. (1988). Transmission of the human immunodeficiency virus: An updated review. International Nursing Review, 35, 44–54.

Fullilove, M. T. (1989). Anxiety and stigmatizing aspects of HIV infection. Journal of Clinical Psychiatry, 50(Suppl.), 6–8.

Gayle, J. A., Selik, R. M., & Chu, S. Y. (1990). Surveillance for AIDS and HIV infection among black and Hispanic children and women of childbearing age, 1981–1989. Morbidity and Mortality Weekly Report, 39(SS-3), 23–30.

Gerberding, J. L. (1988). Occupational health issues for providers of care to patients with HIV infection. Infectious Disease Clinics of North America, 2, 321–328.

Girard, T. M., Pocidolo, J. J., & Murray, J. F. (1991). Primary prophylaxis against common infectious diseases in persons with human immunodeficiency virus infection. American Review of Respiratory Disease, 143, 447–450.

Glass, R. M. (1988). AIDS and suicide. Journal of the American Medical Association, 259, 1369–1370.

Gomatos, P. J., Stamatos, N. M., & Schooley, R. T. (1992). Soluble CD4 immunomodulators, immunotoxins, and other approaches to anti-HIV therapy. In V. T. DeVita, Jr., S. Hellman, & S. A. Rosenberg (Eds.), AIDS: Etiology, diagnosis treatment, and prevention (3rd ed., pp. 406–415). Philadelphia: Lippincott.

Gottlieb, M. S., Schroff, R., Schandker, H. M., Weisman, J. D., Peng, T. F., Wolf, R. A., & Saxon, A. (1981). *Pneumocystis carinii* pneumonia and mucosal candidiasis in previously healthy homosexual men: Evidence of a new acquired cellular immunodeficiency. New England Journal of Medicine, 305, 1425–1431.

Govoni, L. A. (1988). Psychosocial issues of AIDS in the nursing care of homosexual men and their significant others. Nursing Clinics of North America, 23, 749–765.

Grady, C. (1989). Ethical issues in providing nursing care to human immunodeficiency virus-infected populations. Nursing Clinics of North America, 24, 523–534.

Grant, I. H., & Armstrong, D. (1988). Fungal infections in AIDS: Cryptococcosis. Infectious Disease Clinics of North America, 2, 457–464.

Greenspan, J. S., Greenspan, D., & Winkler, J. R. (1990). Diagnosis and management of oral manifestations of HIV infection and AIDS. In M. A. Sande & P. E. Volberding (Eds.), The medical management of AIDS (2nd ed., pp. 131–144). Philadelphia: Saunders.

Grieco, M. H., Lange, M., Buimouici-Klein, E., & Reddy, M. M. (1988). Open study of AL-721 treatment of HIV-infected subjects with generalized lymphadenopathy syndrome: An eight week open trial and follow-up. Antiretroviral Research, 9, 177–190.

Grossman, M. (1988). Children with AIDS. In M. A. Sande & P. A. Volberding (Eds.), The medical management of AIDS (pp. 319–329). Philadelphia: Saunders.

Guinan, M. E., & Hardy, A. (1987). Epidemiology of AIDS in women in the United States: 1981–1986. Journal of the American Medical Association, 257, 2039–2042.

Hammer, J. (1988, August 15). Inside the illegal AIDS drug trade: Mixing greed and good. Newsweek, pp. 41–42.

Helms amendment dropped from bill. (1991, November/December). American Nurse, p. 26.

Hendry, R. M., & Quinnan, G. V., Jr. (1989). Vaccines for the prevention of AIDS. In M. S. Gottlieb, D. J. Jeffries, D. Mildvan, A. J. Pinching, T. C. Quinn, & R. A. Weiss (Eds.), Current topics in AIDS (Vol. 2, pp. 121–149). New York: Wiley.

Henry, O. M., & Hinshaw, A. S. (1989). Foreword. In T. P. Phillips & D. Bloch (Eds.), Nursing and the HIV epidemic: A national action agenda (Proceedings of an invitational workshop, pp. 7–8). Washington, DC: U. S. Department of Health and Human Services.

HIV positives: Data now support reinfection theory. (1991, August). HIV Frontline, p. 4.

Ho, D. D., Pomerantz, R. J., & Kaplan, J. C. (1987). Pathogenesis of infection with human immunodeficiency virus. New England Journal of Medicine, 317(5), 278–286.

Holland, J. C., & Tross, S. (1985). The psychosocial and neuropsychiatric sequelae of the acquired immunodeficiency syndrome and related disorders. Annals of Internal Medicine, 103, 760–764.

Howe, M. (1991a, November 8). Why we're changing from IVDU to IDU. AIDS Information Newsletter, San Francisco VA Medical Center, p. 5.

Howe, M. (1991b, November 22). 1992 Revised classification system for HIV infected and expanded AIDS surveillance case definition for adolescents and adults. AIDS Information Newsletter, San Francisco VA Medical Center, p. 1.

Howe, M. (1991c, December 6). 566C80 receives treatment IND status for AIDS related use. AIDS Information Newsletter, San Francisco VA Medical Center, p. 3.

Howe, M. (1991d, December 20). AZT effectiveness with minorities and women, new analysis shows. AIDS Information Newsletter, San Francisco VA Medical Center, p. 1.

Howe, M. (1992a, January 3). Occupational exposure to bloodborne pathogens: Final rule. AIDS Information Newsletter, San Francisco VA Medical Center, p. 1.

Howe, M. (1992b, November 13). Itraconazole approved. AIDS Information Newsletter, San Francisco VA Medical Center, p. 2.

Hoy, J., Mijch, A., Sandland, M., Grayson, L., Lucas, R., & Dwyer, B. (1990). Quadruple-drug therapy for *Mycobacterium avium-intracellulare* bacteremia in AIDS patients. Journal of Infectious Diseases, 161, 801–805.

Hughes, W. T., McNabb, P. C., Makres, T. D., & Feldman, S. (1974). Efficacy of trimethoprim and sulfamethoxazole in the prevention and treatment of *Pneumocystis carinii* pneumonitis. Antimicrobial Agents and Chemotherapy, 5, 289–293.

Jackson, M. M., Lynch, P., McPherson, D. C., Cummings, M. J., & Greenwalt, N. C. (1987). Why not treat all body substances as infectious? American Journal of Nursing, 87, 1137–1139.

Jacobson, M. A. (1988). Mycobacterial diseases: Tuberculosis and *Mycobacterium avium* complex. Infectious Disease Clinics of North America, 2, 465–474.

Johnston, M. I., & McGowan, J. J. (1992). Strategies and progress in the prevention of antiretroviral agents. In V. T. De Vita, Jr., S. Hellman, & S. A. Rosenberg (Eds.), AIDS: Etiology, diagnosis, treatment, and prevention (3rd ed., pp. 357–371). Philadelphia: Lippincott.

Kanki, P. J., Kurth, R., Becker, W., Dreesman, G., McLane, M.F., & Essex, M. (1985). Antibodies to simian T-lymphotrophic retrovirus type III in African green monkeys, and recognition of STLV-III viral proteins by AIDS and related sera. Lancet, 1, 1330–1332.

Kaplan, L. D. (1988). AIDS-associated lymphomas. Infectious Disease Clinics of North America, 2, 525–532.

Kaposi, M. (1872). Idiopathisches multiples pigment sarcom der haut. Archives of Dermatology and Syphilogie, 4, 265–272.

Katzin, L. (1990). AZT finally approved for pediatric use. American Journal of Nursing, 90, 18.

Kelly, J. A., & St. Lawrence, J. S. (1987). Cautions about condoms in prevention of AIDS. Lancet, 1, 323.

Klug, R. M. (1986). Children with AIDS. American Journal of Nursing, 86, 1126–1131.

Kovacs, J. A., & Masur, H. (1988). Opportunistic infections. In V. T. De Vita, Jr., S. Hellman, & S. A. Rosenberg (Eds.), AIDS: Etiology, diagnosis, treatment, and prevention (2nd ed., pp. 199–225). Philadelphia: Lippincott.

Krigel, R. L., & Friedman-Kien, A. E. (1988). Kaposi's sarcoma in AIDS: Diagnosis and treatment. In V. T. De Vita, Jr., S. Hellman, & S. A. Rosenberg (Eds.), AIDS: Etiology, diagnosis, treatment, and prevention (2nd ed., pp. 245–261). Philadelphia: Lippincott.

Krigel, R. L., Laubenstein, L. J., & Muggia, F. (1983). Kaposi's sarcoma: A new staging classification. Cancer Treatment Reports, 67, 351.

Krim, M. (1986). In M. D. Witt (Ed.), AIDS and patient management: Legal, ethical, and social issues [A Tufts University conference]. Washington, DC: National Health Publishing.

Kubler-Ross, R. (1969). On death and dying. New York: Macmillan.

LaCamera, J. J., Masur, H., & Henderson, D. K. (1985). The acquired immunodeficiency syndrome. Nursing Clinics of North America, 20, 241–257.

LaMontague, J. R., & Myers, M. W. (1987). AIDS: Information on AIDS for the practicing physician. Chicago: American Medical Association.

Laubenstein, L. J. (1984). Staging and treatment of Kaposi's sarcoma in patients with AIDS. In A. E. Friedman-Kien, & L. J. Laubenstein (Eds.), AIDS: The epidemic of Kaposi's sarcoma and opportunistic infections (pp. 51–56). New York: Masson.

Lauerman, J. (1989). Natural history study of pediatric AIDS uncovers new findings. AIDS Patient Care, 3(3), 21–22.

Leonard, R., Zagury, D., Desportes, I., & Bernard, J. (1988). Cytopathic effect of human immunodeficiency virus in T-4 cells is linked to the last stage of virus infection. Proceedings of the National Academy of Sciences of the United States of America, 85, 3570–3574.

Levy, J. A. (1988). The human immunodeficiency virus and its pathogenesis. Infectious Disease Clinics of North America, 2, 285–297.

Levy, J. A., Kaminsky, L. S., & Morrow, W. J. W. (1985). Infection by the retrovirus associated with the acquired immunodeficiency syndrome. Annals of Internal Medicine, 103, 694.

Lewis, K. D., & Thompson, H. B. (1989). Infants, children, and adolescents. In J. H. Flaskerud (Ed.), AIDS/HIV infection: A reference guide for nursing professionals (pp. 111–127). Philadelphia: Saunders.

Lieberman, J. C. (1988). Home health care and hospice for people with HIV infection. In G. Gee & T. A. Moran (Eds.), AIDS: Concepts in nursing practice (pp. 280–303). Baltimore: Williams & Wilkins.

Liebowitz, R. E. (1989). Sociodemographic distribution of AIDS. In J. H. Flaskerud (Ed.), AIDS/HIV infection: A reference guide for nursing professionals (pp. 32–33). Philadelphia: Saunders.

Lifson, A. R. (1988). Do alternate modes of transmission of human immunodeficiency virus exist? A review. Journal of the American Medical Association, 359, 1353–1356.

Little, J., Long, A., & Kehoe, K. B. (1990). AIDS home health, attendant and hospice care pilot project. PAAC Notes, 2(1), 32–56.

Lloyd, J. (1990). Occupational safety guidelines for HIV and other bloodborne pathogens. California AIDS Update, 3, 31–33.

Location of US AIDS clinical trials. (1991). AIDS Clinical Care, 3(3), 1.

MacIntyre, R., Tueller, B., & Wishon, S. L. (1988). Nursing care plans for people with HIV infection. In G. Gee & T. A. Moran (Eds.), AIDS: Concepts in nursing practice (pp. 215–258). Baltimore: Williams & Wilkins.

Mann, J. M. (1989). AIDS: A worldwide pandemic. In M. S. Gottlieb, D. J. Jeffries, D. Mildvan, A. J. Pinching, T. C. Quinn, & R. A. Weiss (Eds.), Current topics in AIDS (Vol. 2, pp. 1–10). New York: Wiley.

Marion, R. W., Wiznia, A. A., Hutcheon, R. G., & Rubinstein, A. (1987). Fetal AIDS syndrome score: Correlation between severity of dysmorphism and age at diagnosis of immunodeficiency. American Journal of Disease Control, 14(4), 429–431.

Markus, K. (1991, November/December). New law requires patient information on advance directives. California Nurse, pp. 8–9.

Martin, J. L., & Vance, C. S. (1984). Behavioral and psychosocial factors in AIDS. American Psychologist, 39, 1303–1308.

Mason, J. O. (1992). A national agenda for women's health. Journal of the American Medical Association, 267, 482.

Masur, H., Michelis, M. A., Greene, J. B., Onorato, I., Uande Stouwe, R. A., Holzman, R. S., Wormser, G., Brettman, L., Lange, M., Murray, M. H., & Cunningham-Rundles, S. (1981). An outbreak of community-acquired *Pneumocystis carinii* pneumonia: Initial manifestations of cellular immune dysfunction. New England Journal of Medicine, 305, 1431–1438.

McKusick, L., & Tafoya, T. (1988, December). Steps to survival: Cross-cultural healing elements in treatment of AIDS. Paper presented at the Kinsey Institute Conference, Bloomington, IN.

McMahon, K. M. (1988). The integration of HIV testing and counseling into nursing practice. Nursing Clinics of North America, 23, 803–821.

Melton, G. B. (1988). Ethical and legal issues in AIDS-related practice. American Psychologist, 43, 941–947.

Mendez, H. (1990). Ambulatory care of infants and children born to HIV-infected mothers. Pediatric Annals, 19, 439–447.

Meng, T. C., Fischl, M. A., Boota, A. M., Spector, S. A., Bennett, D., Bassiakos, Y., Lai, S., Wright, F., & Richman, D. D. (1992). Combination therapy with zidovudine and dideoxycytidine in patients with advanced human immunodeficiency virus infection. Annals of Internal Medicine, 116, 13–20.

Mildvan, D., Mathur, U., Enlow, R. W., Romain, P. L., Winchester, R. J., Colp, C., Singman, H., Adlesberg, B. R., & Spigland, I. (1982). Opportunistic infections and immune deficiency in homosexual men. Annals of Internal Medicine, 96(Part I), 700–704.

Mildvan, D., & Richman, D. D. (1989). Strategies for the treatment of human immunodeficiency virus infection. In M. S. Gottlieb, D. J. Jeffries, D. Mildvan, A. J. Pinching, T. C. Quinn, & R. A. Weiss (Eds.), Current topics in AIDS (Vol. 2, pp. 235–262). New York: Wiley.

Minamoto, G., & Armstrong, D. (1988). Fungal infections in AIDS: Histoplasmosis and coccidioidomycosis. Infectious Disease Clinics of North America, 2, 447–456.

Minkoff, H. L., & DeHovitz, J. A. (1991). Care of women infected with the human immunodeficiency virus. Journal of the American Medical Association, 266, 2253–2258.

Mitsuyasu, R. T. (1988). Kaposi's sarcoma in the acquired immunodeficiency syndrome. Infectious Disease Clinics of North America, 2, 511–523.

Montaner, J. S. G., Lawson, L. M., Levitt, N., Belzberg, A., Schechter, M. T., & Ruedy, J. (1990). Corticosteroids prevent early deterioration in patients with moderately severe *Pneumocystis carinii* pneumonia and the acquired immunodeficiency syndrome (AIDS). Annals of Internal Medicine, 113, 15.

Moon, M. W. (1986). Acquired immunodeficiency syndrome: An update. Journal of Emergency Nursing, 12, 291–293.

Moran, T. A. (1988). Cancers in HIV infection. In G. Gee & T. A. Moran (Eds.), AIDS: Concepts in nursing practice (p. 129). Baltimore: Williams & Wilkins.

Morgan, W. M., & Curran, J. W. (1986). Acquired immunodeficiency virus in the United States: Current and future trends. U.S. Public Health Reports, 101, 459.

Morgan, M., Curran, J. W., & Berkelman, R. L. (1990). The future course of AIDS in the United States. Journal of the American Medical Association, 263, 1539–1540.

Morin, S. F., Charles, K. A., & Malyon, A. K. (1984). The psychological impact of AIDS on gay men. American Psychologist, 39, 1288–1293.

Moss, A. R., Bacchetti, P., Osmond, D., & Kampf, W. (1988). Seropositivity for HIV and the development of AIDS or AIDS related condition: Three-year follow up of the San Francisco General Hospital cohort. British Medical Journal, 296, 745–750.

Namir, S. (1986). Treatment issues concerning persons with AIDS. In L. McKusick (Ed.), What to do about AIDS. Los Angeles: University of California Press.

Namir, S., Wolcott, D. L., Fawzy, F. I., & Alumbaugh, M. J. (1987). Coping with AIDS: Psychological and health implications. Journal of Applied Social Psychology, 17, 309–328.

Nary, G., & Chalice, J. (1992). Defusing a global time bomb. PAAC Notes, 4, 190–192.

National Gay Rights Advocates. (1986). AIDS practice manual: A legal and educational guide. San Francisco: National Gay Rights Advocates and Natural Lawyers Guild.

New OSHA guidelines address HIV and HBV. (1992, January). California Nurse, p. 2.

Newlin, B., & Stringari, S. (1988). Fungal diseases in HIV infection. In G. Gee & T. A. Moran (Eds.), AIDS: Concepts in nursing practice (pp. 177–193). Baltimore: Williams & Wilkins.

Nicholas, S. W., Sondheimer, D. L., Willoughby, A. D., Yaffe, S. J., & Katz, S. L. (1989). Human immunodeficiency virus infection in childhood, adolescence, and pregnancy: A status report and nations research agenda. Pediatrics, 38, 293–307.

Nichols, S. E. (1985). Psychosocial reactions of persons with the acquired immunodeficiency syndrome. Annals of Internal Medicine, 103, 765–767.

NIH provides funding for AIDS research. (1987, November 23). Chemical and Engineering News, p. 2.

Novello, A. C., Wise, P. H., Willoughby, A., & Pizzo, P. A. (1989). Final report of the United States Department of Health and Human Services secretary's work group on pediatric human immunodeficiency virus infection and disease: Content and implications. Pediatrics, 84, 547–555.

Nyamathi, A. M., & Hedderman, M. (1989). Community issues. In J. H. Flaskerud (Ed.), AIDS/HIV infection: A reference guide for nursing professionals (pp. 198–214). Philadelphia: Saunders.

O'Dell, V. C., & Zender, K. D. (1988). Viral diseases in HIV infection. In G. Gee & T. A. Moran (Eds.), AIDS: concepts in nursing practice (pp. 194–212). Baltimore: Williams & Wilkins.

O'Dowd, M. A., & Zofnass, J. S. (1991, October). Psychosocial issues and HIV: Part I. AIDS Clinical Care, 3, 73–75.

O'Grady, S. M., & Frasier, K. E. (1992). Recognizing and managing mycobacterial diseases in clients with AIDS. Nurse Practitioner, 17(9), 41–45.

Office of AIDS (1990). National case summary. California HIV/AIDS Update, 5, 56.

Padian, N. S., Shiboski, S. C., & Jewell, N. P. (1990). The effect of the number of exposures on the risk of heterosexual HIV transmission. Journal of Infectious Diseases, 161, 883–887.

Padian, N. S., Shiboski, S. C., & Jewell, N. P. (1991). Female-to-male transmission of human immunodeficiency virus. Journal of the American Medical Association, 266, 1664–1667.

Pantaleo, G., Graziosi, C., & Fauci, A. S. (1993). The immunopathogenesis of human immunodeficiency virus infection. New England Journal of Medicine, 238, 327–335.

Pape, J. W. (1988). Treatment of gastrointestinal infections. AIDS, 2(Suppl. 1), S161–S167.

Pasnau, R. O. (1989). Anxiety: The silent partner. Journal of Clinical Psychiatry, 50(Suppl. 11), 3–8.

Peterman T. A., & Curran, J. W. (1986). Sexual transmission of human immunodeficiency virus. Journal of the American Medical Association, 256, 2222–2226.

Pitchenik, A. E. (1988). The treatment and prevention of mycobacterial disease in patients with HIV infection. AIDS, 2(Suppl. 1), S177–S182.

Polis, M. A., & Masur, H. (1989). Recent developments in the management of opportunistic infections. In M. S. Gottlieb, D. J. Jeffries, D. Mildvan, A. J. Pinching, T. C. Quinn, & R. A. Weiss (Eds.), Current topics in AIDS (Vol. 2, pp. 207–233). New York: Wiley.

Poole, L. E. (1988). Women and HIV infection. In G. Gee & T. A. Moran (Eds.), AIDS: Concepts in nursing practice (pp. 25–40). Baltimore: Williams & Wilkins.

Porcher, F. K. (1992). HIV-infected pregnant women and their infants. Nurse Practitioner, 17(11), 46–54.

Pratt, R. J. (1986). AIDS: A strategy for nursing care. London: Edward Arnold.

Price, R. W., Brew, B. J., & Roke, M. (1992). Central and peripheral nervous system complications of HIV-1 infection and AIDS. In V. T. DeVita, Jr., S. Hellman, & S. A. Rosenberg (Eds.), AIDS: Etiology, diagnosis, treatment, and prevention (3rd ed., pp. 237–257). Philadelphia: Lippincott.

Primary prophylaxis in HIV-infected patients [Practical briefings]. (1991). Patient Care, 25(10), 12.

Public education defuses cry for forced HIV testing (1991, November/December). California Nurse, p.3.

Redfield, R. R., Wright, D. C., & Fremont, E. C. (1986). The Walter Reed staging system for HTLV-III/LAV infection. New England Journal of Medicine, 314, 131–132.

Remington, J. S., & Araujo, F. G. (1992). A personal approach to toxoplasmosis antimicrobials and immunomodulators for the management of AIDS patients with toxoplasmosis encephalitis. PAAC Notes, 4, 327–331.

Richman, D. D. (1988a). The treatment of HIV infection. AIDS, 2(Suppl. 1), S137–142.

Richman, D. D. (1988b). The treatment of HIV infection: Azidothymidine (AZT) and other new antiviral drugs. Infectious Disease Clinics of North America, 2, 397–405.

Richman, D. D., Fischl, M. A., Grieco, M. H., & Gottlieb, M. S. (1987). The toxicity of azidothymidine (AZT) in the treatment of patients with AIDS and AIDS-related complex: A double-blind, placebo-controlled trial. New England Journal of Medicine, 317, 192–197.

Robertson, J. A. (1983). The rights of the critically ill. Cambridge, MA: Ballinger.

Salisbury, D. M. (1986). AIDS: Psychosocial implications. Journal of Psychosocial Nursing, 24(12), 13–16.

Sanchez, L. (1992, October 12). Pacto reaches out in Spanish for Latinos threatened by AIDS. San Diego Union, p. B1.

Sande, M. A., & Volberding, P. A. (1992). The medical management of AIDS (3rd ed.). Philadelphia: Saunders.

Schechter, M. T., Craib, K. J. P., Le, T. N., Montaner, J. S. G., Douglas, B., Sestak, P., Willoughby, B., & O'Shaughnessy, M. V. (1990). Susceptibility to AIDS progression appears early in HIV infection. AIDS, 4, 185–190.

Schietinger, H. (1986). A home care plan for AIDS. American Journal of Nursing, 86, 1020–1028.

Sedaka, S. D., & O'Reilly, M. (1986). The financial implications of AIDS. Caring, 5(6), 38–46.

Selwyn, P. A. (1986a). AIDS: What is now known: I. History and immunovirology. Hospital Practice, 21(4), 67–83.

Selwyn, P. A. (1986b). AIDS: What is now known: II. Epidemiology. Hospital Practice, 21(6), 127–164.

Selwyn, P. A. (1986c). AIDS: What is now known: IV. Psychosocial aspects, treatment prospects. Hospital Practice, 21(10), 125–164.

Signs and symptoms associated with HIV infection in children. (1991). AIDS Clinical Care, 3(4), 1.

Stanhope, M., Sheahan, S., & Kent, E. (1984). The community health nurse as client care coordinator-collaborator. In M. Stanhope & J. Lancaster (Eds.), Community health nursing: Process and practice for promoting health (pp. 744–761). St. Louis: Mosby.

Statistics from the World Health Organization and the Centers for Disease Control. (1990). AIDS, 4, 375–379.

Stern, M. (1990, June 25). Decay of the underclass mauls its children. San Diego Union, pp. A1, A5.

Task Force on Pediatric AIDS. (1989). Infants and children with acquired immunodeficiency syndrome: Placement in adoption and foster care. Pediatrics, 83, 609–612.

Thurber, F., & Berry, B. (1990). Children with AIDS: Issues and future directions. Journal of Pediatric Nursing, 5, 168–178.

Tozzi, V., Bordi, E., Galgani, S., Leoni, G. C., Narciso, P., Sette, P., & Visco, G. (1989.) Fluconazole treatment of cryptococcosis in patients with acquired immune deficiency syndrome. American Journal of Medicine, 87, 353.

Tross, S., & Hirsch, D. A. (1988). Psychological distress and neuropsychological complications of HIV infection and AIDS. American Psychologist, 43, 929–934.

Ungvarski, P. J. (1989). Nursing management of the adult client. In J. H. Flaskerud (Ed.), AIDS/HIV infection: A reference guide for nursing professionals (pp. 74–110). Philadelphia: Saunders.

Vella, S., Guilian, M., Pezzotti, P., et al. (1992). Survival of zidovudine-treated patients with AIDS compared with that of contemporary untreated patients. Journal of the American Medical Association, 267, 1232–1236.

Vogt, M. W., Hartshorn, K. L., Furman, P. A., & Chou, T. C. (1987). Ribavirin antagonizes the effect of azidothymidine on HIV replication. Science, 235, 1376–1379.

Volberding, P. A. (1988). Treatment of malignant disease in AIDS patients. AIDS, 2(Suppl. 1), S169–S175.

Wesorick, B. (1990). Standards of nursing care: A model for clinical practice. Philadelphia: Lippincott.

Williams, A. B. (1992). The epidemiology, clinical manifestations, and health-maintenance needs of women infected with HIV. Nurse Practitioner, 17(5), 27–41.

Williams P. (1991). A new focus on AIDS in women. ASM News, 57, 130–134.

Wilson, S., & Lein, B. (1992, Summer/Fall). HIV disease in women. Treatment Issues, 6(7[Special Edition]), 1–25.

Wishon, S. L., & Gee, G. (1988). Children and HIV infection. In G. Gee & T. A. Moran (Eds.), AIDS: Concepts in nursing practice (pp. 41–61). Baltimore: Williams & Wilkins.

Wiznia, A., & Rubinstein, A. (1988). Pediatric infections and therapy. AIDS, 2(Suppl. 1), S195–S199.

Wofsy, C. B. (1987). Human immunodeficiency virus infection in women. Journal of the American Medical Association, 257, 2074–2076.

Wofsy, C. B. (1988). Prevention of HIV transmission. Infectious Disease Clinics of North America, 2, 307–319.

Wofsy, C. B. (1992). Therapeutic issues in women with HIV disease. In M. A. Sande & P. A. Volberding (Eds.), The medical management of AIDS (3rd ed., pp. 465–476). Philadelphia: Saunders.

Wolcott, D. L. (1986). Psychosocial aspects of acquired immune deficiency syndrome and the primary care physician. Annals of Allergy, 57, 95–101.

Wolfe, P. (1989). Clinical manifestations and treatment. In J. H. Flaskerud (Ed.), AIDS/HIV infection: A reference guide for nursing professionals (pp.58–73). Philadelphia: Saunders.

World Health Organization. (1992). AIDS statistical information as of January 1, 1993. Medline, Computer Information Service.

Wormser, G. P., Stahl, R. E., & Buttone, E. J. (1987). AIDS: Acquired immune deficiency syndrome and other manifestations of HIV infection. Park Ridge, NJ: Noyes.

Yap, P. L. (1990). The uses of intravenous immunoglobulin (IVIG) in the management of HIV infection in the pediatric population. PAAC Notes, 2, 71–73.

Yarandi, H. N., & Simpson, S. H. (1991). The logistic regression model and the odds of testing HIV positive. Nursing Research, 40, 372–373.

INDEX

A

ABGs, 92, 93
Abstinence, 28
Acquired immune deficiency syndrome (AIDS). *See* AIDS
Acute HIV syndrome, 9
Acyclovir (Zovirax), 106-108
Adolescents,
    AIDS epidemiology and demographics, 65
        assessment and treatment of, 66
        education of, 66-67
        psychosocial issues of, 66
        serologic testing and diagnosis of, 65-66
Advance directives, 182, 188
Advocacy, 180-181
African Kaposi's sarcoma, 110-111
AIDS,
    CDC Definition of, 3, 9, 13-17, 51
    defined, 12, 197
    demographics of, 3-5, 65
    ethical issues, 180-183
    first appearance of, 2
    legal issues, 183-190
    management of symptoms, 157-158
    mandatory reporting of diagnosis, 186
    progression from asymptomatic HIV disease, 10-11
    psychosocial issues, 165-176
    women and, 40-45
    See also HIV; Opportunistic infections
AIDS clinical trials units (ACTUs), 74, 81
AIDS dementia complex (ADC), 115-117, 160
AIDS-related complex (ARC), 9, 197
AL-721, 75
Ambulatory care, 159-160
Amikacin (Amikin), 103
Amphotericin B,
    used for candidiasis, 98
    used for coccidioidomycosis, 87
    used for *cryptococcus neoformans*, 99
    used for histoplasmosis, 100

Ampligen, 78
ANA Code of Ethics, 174-175, 180
Anal intercourse, 21, 23
    See also Sexual intercourse
Anergy, 101
Ann Arbor staging system, 113
Anorexia, 157
Ansamycin, 103
Antibody, 197
Antiemetics, 94
Antigen, 197
Antigenemia, 197
Antimicrobial therapy, 93
Antiviral, 197
Anxiety, 126, 157, 169
Assessments,
    in adolescents, 66
    for disability, 160
    for home health care, 154-155
    in hospital and home setting, 64-65
    of infants and children, 54-56
    of patient symptoms, 123-124
    of persons with HIV disease, 86-87
    psychosocial, 170-172
    of women with AIDS, 41-42
    See also Nursing care
Atovaquone (Mepron), 93, 94
Autologous transfusions, 24
Autonomy, 180-181
Azidothymidine [AZT], Retrovir. *See* Zidovudine (azidothymidine [AZT], Retrovir)
AZT. *See* Zidovudine (azidothymidine [AZT], Retrovir)

B

Bacterial opportunistic infections,
    listed, 90
    mycobacterium avium complex (MAC), 102-104

mycobacterium avium-intracellulare (MAI), 102-104
mycobacterium tuberculosis, 101-102
salmonellosis, 104-105
shigellosis, 105
staphylococcus aureus, 104
See also Opportunistic infections
Bacterium, 197
Barrier equipment, 32-33
B cell, 6, 197
B-cell lymphoma, 114
Beneficence, 181, 182
Biaxin, 103
Biopsy, 197
Blood glucose levels, 94
Blood products,
    HIV infection through, 20, 22
    OSHA blood-borne pathogen standard, 35
    screening, 23-24
"The Blood Donor Information Form," 184
Blood urea nitrogen (BUN), 99
Brain lymphomas, 53
Burkitt's lymphoma, 114

C

California Collaborative Treatment Group (CCTG), 74
Candida esophagitis, 42, 97
Candidiasis, 58, 96-98, 197
Case management, 148
CD4 T cells,
    combination therapy and, 79-80
    count as AIDS criteria, 12
    during HIV disease, 9
    HIV-induced response of, 6-8
    level in children, 53
    PCP treatment and, 94-95
    treatment decisions and, 87
    virus-receptor inhibitors and, 74-75
    See also Helper/inducer T cells
CD8 cells. See Suppressor T cells (CD8)
CDC,
    HIV disease definition in children, 50
    HIV infection diagnosis in children, 49
    HIV prevention recommendations by, 32-34
    immunization recommendations, 61, 63
    mandatory reporting of AIDS to, 186
    staging system, 11
    zidovudine recommendations by, 34-35
CDC Definition of AIDS,
    changes in, 3
    described, 13-17
    illnesses designated as AIDS-defining criteria, 9
    inclusion of cervical cancer in, 42
    revised, 51
Cell-medicated immunity, 197
Centers for Disease Control (CDC). See CDC
Cervical cancer, 42
Cervical dysplasia, 42
Cervical neoplasia, 42
Chemotherapy,
    for Kaposi's sarcoma, 112-113
    See also Drug therapy
Children,
    AIDS epidemiology of, 48-49
    definition of HIV disease in, 50
    diagnostic evaluation of, 54-55
    education for, 64
    HIV disease in adults vs., 52-53
    HIV disease classification in, 50-52
    HIV disease manifestations in, 53-54
    HIV infection classification system in, 52
    HIV infection diagnosis criteria for, 49
    immune systems in, 49-50
    immunizations for, 61, 63
    medical management of, 56-61
    nursing care for, 64-65
    transmission to, 23
Ciprofloxacin, 103
Clarithromycin (Biaxin), 103
Classic Kaposi's sarcoma, 110-111
Class P-1, 50
Class P-2, 50
Class P-O, 50
Clindamycin, 94, 95
Clofazamine, 103
Clotrimazole (Gyne-Lotrimin), 97, 98
Clotrimazole (Mycelex) troches, 97
CMV infection, 108-109

Coccidioides immitis, 100
Coccidioidomycosis, 100-101
Code of Ethics (ANA), 174-175, 180
Cofactor, 197
Combination therapy, 79-80
Compliance, 160
Compound Q, 79
Condoms, 28, 29-30, 44
Confidentiality, 182-186
Conservators, 187
Contextualization, 173
Coping, 171
Cough, 127, 157
Counseling, 184
Cryptococcus neoformans, 58
Cryptosporidium, 57
Culdoscopy, 42
Cunnilingus, 29
Cytomegalovirus, 59, 108-109
Cytotoxic T cells, 6

D

D4T, 77-78
Dapsone, 94
DdC, 77
Death,
    nurses's rituals related to, 176
    preparation for, 170
    See also Legal issues
Dementia, 115-117, 160
Denial, 169
Deoxyribonucleic acid (DNA), 6
Depression, 128, 157, 160, 168-169
Dextran sulfate, 73-75
Diagnosis, 198
Diagnosis-related groups (DRGs), 149
Diarrhea, 61, 129, 157
Didanosine, 76-77
Dideoxycitidine (ddC), 73, 87
Dideoxyinosine (ddI), 73, 87
Diflucan, 87
Diphenhydramine hydrochloride (Benadryl), 94
Directives to physicians, 188
Discharge planning,
    described, 148-151
    example of, 151-152
Disclosure, 184-186
DNA (deoxyribonucleic acid), 198
Drug resistance, 198
Drug therapy,
    assessment for, 87
    for *Candida albicans,* 97-98
    for children, 56-61
    for CMV infections, 109
    for coccidioidomycosis, 101
    combination, 79-80
    compound Q, 79
    for *cryptosporidium,* 57, 96
    for herpes zoster or varicella-zoster virus, 107-108
    for histoplasmosis, 100
    immunotherapy, 79
    inhibitors of reverse transcriptase, 76-78
    interferon, 79
    Kaposi's sarcoma, 111-113
    for lymphoma, 114
    for MAC and MAI, 103
    for MTB, 102
    for PCP, 93-94
    research on HIV, 72-74
    ribavirin (Virazole), 78-79
    for salmonellosis, 105
    shigellosis, 105
    for *staphylococcus aureus,* 104
    for *toxoplasma gondii,* 57, 96
    vaccines, 80-81
    virus-receptor inhibitors, 74-75
    See also Treatment; Zidovudine (azidothymidine [AZT], Retrovir)
Durable power of attorney, 182, 187-188
Durable power of attorney for health care, 188
Dysphagia, 138

E

Edema, 130
Education,
    of adolescents, 66-67
    of children and parents, 64
    as preventive measure, 28

regarding Patient Self Determination Act, 188
on safe sexual practices, 28-30
to change behaviors, 185
topics listed for AIDS, 161-162
for women, 44
"Eggs-Act," 75
Emotional arousal, 173
Enzyme-linked immunosorbent assay (ELISA), 184, 198
"Epidemiologic Aspects" (*The New England Journal of Medicine*), 2
Epidemiology, 198
Epstein-Barr virus (EBV), 11, 198
Erythema multiforme, 95
Ethambutol (Myambutol), 103
Ethical issues, 180-183
Etiology, 198
Executors, 189

F

Fatigue, 131, 153
FDA, 72-73
Fear, 132, 169
Fellatio, 29
Female-to-male transmission, 21, 40
Fever, 133, 157
Finsidar, 95
5-flucytosine (5FC), 99
Fluconazole (Diflucan), 87, 97, 100
Flucytosine, 99
Foscarnet (Foscavir), 78, 106-107, 109
Fungal opportunistic infections,
    Candida albicans, 96-98
    coccidioidomycosis, 100-101
    cryptococcus neoformans, 98-100
    histoplasmosis, 100
    listed, 90
    See also Opportunistic infections

G

Ganciclovir, 109
Gay Men's Health Crisis (GMHC), 29

Gay-related immune deficiency syndrome (GRIDS), 2
Genital ulcers, 42
Genital warts, 42
Genome, 198
"Gray market," 73
Grief, 172
Group rituals, 173
Guilt, 169
Gyne-Lotrimin, 97, 98

H

Hairy leukoplakia, 198
Handwashing, 32
Healing elements, 172-174
Health care setting, 30, 32-34
Health care workers,
    CDC recommendations for, 32-34
    occupational exposure of, 24, 34-36
    the Tarasoff Doctrine duties of, 182-183
    See also Nursing care
Helms Amendment, 35-36
Helper/inducer T cells, 6
    See also CD4 T cells
Helper/suppressor ratio, 198
Hemophilia, 198
Hepatitis B virus (HBV), 11, 20, 24
Hepatomegaly, 198
Herpes simplex viruses (HSV),
    defined, 198
    as opportunistic infection, 105-107
    treatment for, 59
    women with, 42
Herpesviruses, 11
Herpes zoster virus (HZV), 107-108, 198
Heterosexual transmission,
    demographics of, 4
    rise of, 3, 21
HGP-30 vaccine, 80
High-risk behaviors,
    blood transfusions, 22
    defining, 198
    maternal transmission, 23
    sexual, 21
    substance abuse, 22

Histoplasma capsulatum, 100
HIV,
    AIDS development and, 3, 5
    CDC prevention recommendations, 32-34
    described, 5-6, 198
    groups at high risk of, 23-24
    health care workers and, 24, 34-36
    identification of, 2
    life cycle of Type I, 72
    mandatory testing movement, 35-36
    methods of transmission, 20-23
    origins of, 6
    pregnancy and, 43
    preventing transmission of, 28-30
    research progress on, 73-74
    testing for antibodies, 184-185
    transmission risks, 20-21
    See also AIDS
HIV disease,
    in adolescents, 65-67
    adults vs. infants/children, 52-53
    care plans for patients with, 125
    CDC classifications of, 50-52
    in children, 50-54
    clinical trials for treatment of, 72-73
    defined, 198
    drugs for treating, 71-72
    emotional reactions to, 168-170
    individual unique progression of, 11-12
    nursing ethics and, 181-183
    progression of, 8-11
    stages and treatment of, 11-12, 88
    in women, 42-45
    See also Opportunistic infections; Psychosocial issues
Hivid, 77
Home health care, 152-159
    See also Nursing care
Homosexuals,
    AIDS transmission among, 3
    high risk group, 23
    issues confronting AIDS patients, 167
    special legal issues of, 186
HSV-1, 105-106
HSV-2, 105-106
Human immunodeficiency virus (HIV). *See* HIV

Human papillomavirus (HPV), 42
Human T-cell lymphotropic virus type III (HTLV-III), 2
    See also HIV
Humoral immunity, 198
Hyperpigmentation, 103
Hypoglychemia, 94

I

Illness phase, 172
Immune system,
    defining, 198
    description of normal, 6-8
    of infants and children, 49-50
Immunizations, 61, 63
Immunoadhesins, 75
Immunomodulators, 73
Immunotherapy, 79
Immunotoxins, 75
Impaired mobility, 133
Incubation period, 199
Infants,
    AIDS epidemiology in, 48-49
    diagnostic evaluation of, 54-55
    HIV disease in adults vs., 52-53
    HIV disease manifestations in, 53-54
    immune systems in, 49-50
    immunizations for, 61, 63
    medical management of, 56-61
    nursing care for, 64-65
    psychosocial issues, 62
    See also Maternal transmission
Infections, 135
    See also Opportunistic infections
Informed consent, 181
INH, 103
Inhibitors of reverse transcriptase,
    ampligen, 78
    d4T, 77-78
    dideoxycytidine (Zalcitabine, Hivid), 77
    dideoxyinosine (Didanosine, Videx), 76-77
    suramin, 78
    trisodium phosphonoformate (PFA, Foscarnet, Foscavir), 78
    zidovudine (Retrovir) or AZT, 76

Injecting drug user (IDU), 22, 167
Inosine Pranobex (Isoprinosine), 79
Interferon, 79
Inter vivos trust, 187
Intravenous immunoglobulin therapy, 61
In utero transmission. *See* Maternal transmission
In vitro, 199
Isolation, 136, 169
Isoniazid (INH), 103
Isoprinosine, 79
Itraconazole (Sporanox), 87

J

Joint ownership, 186
Joint tenancy, 186

K

Kaposi's sarcoma, 10, 109-113, 199
Karnofsky Scale, 149, 150
Kemron, 79
Ketoconazole (Nizoral), 42, 87, 97-98
Killer T cells. *See* Cytotoxic T cells

L

Latency, 199
Latex condoms, 28, 29-30, 44
Laundry, 33-34
Leakproof containers, 33
Legal issues,
    estate matters, 186-189
    testing consent/confidentiality, 184-185
Lesion, 199
Leukocytes, 7
Life-cycle phase, 172
Living wills, 182, 188
Loss, 172
Lymphadenopathy virus (LAV), 2, 199
    See also HIV
Lymph node (gland), 199
Lymphocytes, 6, 20

Lymphoid interstitial pneumonia, 53
Lymphokines, 6
Lymphomas, 114, 116, 199

M

Macrophages, 6
Macular, 199
Male-to-female transmission, 21, 40
Mandatory testing, 35-36
Maternal transmission,
    chance of, 43
    described, 20, 52-53
    increased rate of, 30
    risk of, 23
    See also Infants
Memory T cells, 6
Mepron, 93
Mismatched RNA, 78
Monoclonal antibodies, 74
Morbidity, 199
Morbidity and Mortality Weekly Report (MMWR), 2
Mortality, 199
    See also Death
Mortality rates, 5
Multiple sexual partners, 21, 29
Myambutol, 103
Mycelex, 97
Mycobacterium avium complex (MAC), 102-104
Mycobacterium avium-intracellulare (MAI), 58, 89, 102-104
Mycobacterium tuberculosis (MTB), 59, 101-102

N

National Institute of Allergy and Infectious Diseases (NIAID), 74
Nausea, 137, 158
Needles, cleaning, 30, 31
Neurosyphilis, 42
Neutropenia, 109
Neutrophils, 6
The New England Journal of Medicine, 2

NIH, 72-73
Nilstat, 97
Nizoral, 87
Non-Hodgkin's lymphoma, 113-114
Nonmaleficence, 181, 182
Nonoxynol-9 spermicide, 28, 29-30, 44
Normative ethics, 180
Nursing care,
    ambulatory, 159-160
    for anxiety, 126
    appropriate attitudes of, 174-175
    for cough, 127, 157
    for depression, 128, 157, 160
    for diarrhea, 129, 157
    for edema, 130
    ethical considerations of, 180-183
    for fatigue, 131
    for fearful patient, 132
    for fever, 133, 158
    for HIV disease patients, 125
    home health care, 152-159
    for impaired mobility, 133
    for infection control, 135
    for isolated patient, 136
    management of, 148
    meeting challenge of, 143
    for nausea and vomiting, 137, 158
    for oral lesions, dysphagia, and odynophagia, 138
    for pain, 139, 158
    planning, 123-124
    process of, 122-123
    role of, 122
    for shortness of breath, 140
    for skin problems, 141
    to manage emotional distress, 172-174
    for wasting, weight loss, 142
    See also Assessments; Discharge planning; Health care workers
Nursing ethics,
    described, 180-181
    HIV infection and, 181-183
Nursing fidelity, 181
Nutritional support, 61
Nutrition education, 162
Nystatin (Nilstat), 97
Nystatin vaginal tablets, 97

O

Occupational exposure, 34-36
    See also Health care workers
Odynophagia, 138
One-hand recapping technique, 33
Opportunistic infections,
    AIDS dementia complex, 115-117
    bacterial infections, 101-105
    described, 87-90, 199
    fungal infections, 96-101
    protozoal infections, 90, 92-96
    treatment of, 91-92
    tumors, 109-116
    types listed, 90
    viral infections, 105-109
Oral contraceptives, 21
Oral herpes infections, 61
Oral intercourse, 23, 29
Oral lesions, 138
Orthostatic hypotension, 199
OSHA blood-borne pathogen standard, 35

P

Pain, 139, 158
Pancytopenia, 199
Pap tests, 42
Papular, 199
Parallel tracking, 73
Parents, education for, 64
Passive immunotherapy, 74
Pathogen, 199
Patients,
    appropriate attitudes toward, 174-175
    care for ambulatory, 159-160
    care plans for HIV disease, 125
    caring for coughing, 127, 157
    caring for isolated, 136
    compliance by, 160
    counseling for, 184
    death of, 170, 176
    depressed, 128, 157, 160
    estate matters, 186-189
    fearful, 132
    fevered, 133, 157

giving informed consent, 181
home health care for, 152-159
with impaired mobility, 133
infection control for, 135
Karnofsky Scale, 149, 150
with oral lesions, dysphagia, and odynophagia, 138
with pain, 139, 157
psychosocial assessment, 170-172
with shortness of breath, 140
signs and symptoms of, 123-124, 157-158
with skin problems, 141
suffering from diarrhea, 129, 157
suffering from edema, 130
suffering from fatigue, 131, 153
suffering with nausea/vomiting, 137, 158
treating for anxiety, 126, 157
wasting, 142
See also Discharge planning
Patient Self Determination Act (1992), 188
Pentam, 94
Pentamidine (Pentam), 94
Peptide T, 75
Personal qualities of healer, 173
PFA, 78
Phagocytic cells, 6
Pneumocystis carinii pneumonia (PCP),
AIDS and, 2
described, 90, 92-93
early cause of death, 10
as opportunistic infection, 89
preventative therapy for, 94-95
side effects of drug therapy for, 94
treatment of, 57, 60, 93
Polymerase chain reaction, 23
Power of attorney, 187
Power of naming, 173
Powers of appointment, 187
PPD converters, 102
Prevention education, 161-162
Primary level nursing care, 122
Primary lymphoma, 114, 116
Project Inform, 74
Prophylaxis,
for cryptococcosis, 99-100
for PCP, 94-95
Protozoal opportunistic infections,

cryptosporidium, 96
listed, 90
Toxoplasma gondii, 57, 95-96
See also Opportunistic infections; *Pneumocystis carinii* pneumonia (PCP)
Proxy designation, 182
Pseudomonas exotoxin, 75
Psychiatric evaluation, 160
Psychosocial issues,
approaches to healing, 172-174
assessment of, 156
emotional reactions to HIV disease, 168-170
for nurses and their families, 175-176
patient assessment, 170-172
sources of, 166-168
in treating adolescents, 66
in treating infants/children, 62
See also Depression
Pulmonary lymphocytic hyperplasia, 53
Punctuation rituals, 173
Pyramidal tract signs, 199
Pyrazinamide, 102
Pyrimethamine, 96

R

Recombinant soluble CD4, 74-75
Retrovirus, 5-6, 199
See also HIV
Reverse transcriptase enzyme, 5-6, 199
Ribavirin (Virazole), 78-79
Ribonucleic acid (RNA), 5
Rifabutin (Ansamycin), 103
Rifampin, 102
Risk factor education, 161
RsCD4IgG1, 75

S

Safe sexual practices, 28-30, 43-44
Salmonellosis, 104-105
Screening laboratory tests,
for adolescents, 65-66
confidentiality of, 185

consent to, 184-185
   establishment of clinics for, 159
   initial, 86
   for PCP diagnosis, 90
   psychological stress of, 166
Secondary level nursing care, 122
Self-esteem, 172
Self-mastery, 173
Septra DS, 94
Seroconversion, 199
Sexual intercourse,
   HIV infection through, 20, 21
   practiced by adolescents, 65
   preventing HIV through, 28-30
   social pressures regarding, 167
   unprotected, 23
Sexual partners,
   AMA disclosure recommendations, 185
   confidentiality principles and, 185-186
   disclosure to, 182-183
Sharp object disposal, 33
Shigellosis, 105
Shingles, 107-108
"Shooting galleries," 22
Shortness of breath, 140
Situational distress, 170
Skin popping, 22
Skin problems, 141
Social support systems, 156, 172
Splenomegaly, 199
Sporanox, 87
Stages of Deterioration: AIDS/ARC Intervention, 11
Staphylococcus aureus, 104
Stevens-Johnson syndrome, 95
STLV-III virus, 6
Subclass A, 50
Subclass B, 50-51
Subclass D, 51
Subclass E, 51-52
Subclass F, 52
Substance abuse,
   cleaning needles, 30, 31
   as high risk behavior, 22
   preventing transmission through, 30
   See also Injecting drug user (IDU)
Suicide, 168-169

Sulfadiazine, 96
Suppressor T cells (CD8), 6
Suramin, 78
Symptomatic HIV disease, 9
   See also HIV disease
Syndrome, 200
Syphilis, 42

T

Tarasoff Doctrine, 182-183
TAT inhibitors, 75
T cells, 6, 200
Teenagers. *See* Adolescents
Tertiary level nursing care, 122
T helper cell, 200
Thrush, 61, 97, 200
TMP/SMX (Septra DS), 94
Toxic epidermal neurolysis, 95
Toxoplasma antibodies, 87
Toxoplasma gondii, 57, 95-96
Transmission education, 161
Treatment,
   of ADC, 117
   of adolescents, 66
   for anxiety, 126
   clinical trials for HIV infection, 72-73
   for coughing, 127, 157
   for depression, 128
   for diarrhea, 128
   for edema, 130
   for fatigue, 131
   of fearful patient, 132
   for fever, 133
   heating HIV infected blood, 81
   of HIV-infected children, 56-61
   for infection, 135
   for lymphoma, 114
   for patient with impaired mobility, 134
   stages of HIV disease, 88
   use of parallel tracking in, 73
   where to get, 81-82
   See also Drug therapy
Trimethoprim, 94
Trusts, 187
T suppressor cell, 200

Tuberculosis, 101-102
Tumors, 10, 109-113, 200

U

U.S. Public Health Service conference (1986), 3

V

Vaccines, 80-81
Vaginal candidiasis, 42, 97, 98
Vaginal intercourse, 23
Varicella-zoster virus (VZV), 59, 107-108, 200
Vesicle, 200
Videx, 76-77
Viral opportunistic infections,
    cytomegalovirus, 108-109
    herpes simplex viruses, 105-107
    herpes zoster or varicella-zoster virus, 107-108
    listed, 90
    See also Opportunistic infections
Virazole, 78-79
Virus, 200
Virus-receptor inhibitors, 74-75
Vomiting, 137, 158

W

Waste disposal, 33
Wasting, 142
Weight loss, 142
Western blot test, 200
WHO immunization recommendations, 61
Wills, 188-189
Women,
    AIDS assessment of, 41-42
    AIDs epidemiology, 40-41
    HIV disease in, 42-43
    pregnancy and HIV in, 43
    safe sex guidelines for, 43-44
    special issues for, 44-45
World Health Organization (WHO), 5

Y

Yeast infections, 42

Z

Zalcitabine, 77
Zidovudine (azidothymidine [AZT], Retrovir),
    approved by FDA, 73
    female vs. male response to, 42-43
    research findings on, 76
    treatment of ADC with, 117
    treatment with, 34-35
    treatment for young children, 60-61
Zovirax, 106-108

PRETEST KEY
NURSING APPROACHES TO HIV/AIDS CARE

1. d   Chapter 1
2. d   Chapter 2
3. d   Chapter 2
4. d   Chapter 3
5. c   Chapter 3
6. c   Chapter 4
7. b   Chapter 4
8. d   Chapter 5
9. c   Chapter 5
10. a Chapter 5
11. d Chapter 5
12. d Chapter 6
13. c Chapter 7
14. d Chapter 7
15. b Chapter 7
16. c Chapter 7
17. c Chapter 8
18. b Chapter 8
19. a Chapter 8
20. a Chapter 9
21. b Chapter 9
22. c Chapter 10
23. d Chapter 10
24. c Chapter 11
25. d Chapter 11

NURSING APPROACHES TO HIV/AIDS CARE

WESTERN SCHOOLS' NURSING CONTINUING EDUCATION
EVALUATION

Instructions: Mark your answers to the following questions with a #2 pencil on the "Student Evaluation" section of your Scantron answer sheet provided with this course. You should not return this sheet. Please use the scale below to rate the following statements:

- **A Agree Strongly**
- **B Agree Somewhat**
- **C Disagree Somewhat**
- **D Disagree Strongly**

1. Described changes in the demographics of HIV infection and how the virus affects the human body and the immune system.

2. Described how HIV is transmitted and indicated which populations are at risk for HIV infection.

3. Described practices that reduce the risk of becoming infected with HIV in the hospital setting and in the social environment.

4. Discussed epidemiologic findings, assessment procedures, and common problems associated with HIV disease in women.

5. Described the differences and similarities between HIV infection and AIDS in adults and in infants and children.

6. Discussed drug and nondrug therapies proposed, being studied, and being used to treat HIV disease.

7. Discussed the opportunistic infections, tumors, and dementia associated with HIV disease and current medical treatments of these disorders.

8. Described nursing care problems of persons infected with HIV, specified appropriate nursing diagnoses and interventions, and showed how to develop a plan of care for these problems.

9. Identified the home care needs of patients with AIDS, specified a discharge plan to meet those needs after hospitalization, and recognized problems in ambulatory care and specified appropriate nursing interventions.

10. Described the psychologic and social issues that affect patients with HIV disease, their care providers, and health care workers.

11. Described the ethical and legal issues associated with HIV disease and specified the role of nurses who care for patients with ethical and legal problems.

The "Student Evaluation" section of the Scantron answer sheet lists 20 evaluation responses. Please ignore 12 through 20. This is a standardized form used for many courses.